Contrast-Enhanced Ultrasound of the Urinary Tract

Giovanni Regine · Maurizio Atzori
Romano Fabbri

Contrast-Enhanced Ultrasound of the Urinary Tract

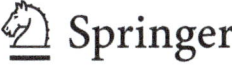

Giovanni Regine
Maurizio Atzori
Romano Fabbri
UOC Radiologia della Piastra
S. Camillo-Forlanini Hospital
Rome
Italy

ISBN 978-88-470-5430-1   ISBN 978-88-470-5432-5 (eBook)
DOI 10.1007/978-88-470-5432-5
Springer Milan Heidelberg New York Dordrecht London

Library of Congress Control Number: 2013937730

The contents of this book are based on: Ecocontrastografia dell'apparato urinario. G. Regine, M. Atzori, R. Fabbri © Springer-Verlag Italia 2012.

Printed on acid-free paper

Springer is part of Springer Science+Business Media (www.springer.com)

Preface

The ever-increasing return to the use of ultrasound contrast media has eliminated, or is in the process of eliminating, a kind of subordination of this method in comparison with other imaging technologies, such as TC or RM, considered to be more accurate, and therefore better for diagnosis. Yet, for a number of years now ultrasound has found its contrast media which, in the form of microbubbles, has given the technique a notable 'effervescence', opening the way for many new tools, both diagnostic and in the future probably also treatments, which were before unthinkable. Following the current growing interest, this paper seeks to analyze the applications of ultrasound using second-generation contrast enhancement for renal pathology, comparing our results with the current publications on the matter. The unique chemical and physical characteristics of the type of contrast chosen, combined with the use of specially designed software which is now standard on most middle-to high-grade ultrasound equipment, appear to be advantageous particularly in the evaluation of ischemic or traumatic pathology and in the characterization of cystic renal lesions. Another application now validated is in the follow-up after a kidney transplant, allowing for the identification of potential early or late complications, when used with perfusion indexes.

The most recent applications include the attempt to identify solid renal lesions and to define the T parameter in the staging of bladder lesions. Uses of the technique that are still 'unofficial' include evaluations of the vesicoureteral reflux in pediatric patients, and in general, all uses in the pediatric field.

The authors, delineating their experience based on a retrospective evaluation of the cases they have seen, hope to have produced something useful for those who have dedicated themselves to the use of microbubbles, or plan to do so, in the daily challenges of diagnostics that await them, whether experts or beginners. They also express their deep gratitude to their colleagues at the "Unità Operativa", in particular Dr. Simonetta Pascoli, untiring proponent of the method, as well as T. S. R. M Carlo Pace for the technological assistance which was vital for the present contribution.

Rome, May 2013

G. Regine
M. Atzori
R. Fabbri

Contents

Introduction

1

1.1 Introduction

One can find many published studies on the use of second-generation ultrasound contrast media (UCM) for kidney disease, but in recent years there have been an increasing number of publications regarding applications for other organs: the kidney, small intestine, pancreas, testes, and prostate [1]. The reason for this shift is in the unique chemical and physical characteristics of the contrast medium employed, which in this case is comprised of sulphur hexafluoride microbubbles with a diameter of 2–5 μm. Because of their size, once introduced into the blood stream they cannot be diffused into extravascular spaces. Thus, they take on similar characteristics to blood-pool contrast media, with the difference that they can pass through the pulmonary alveolar-capillary membrane and therefore be disposed of primarily through the respiratory process. This means of elimination makes second-generation CM recommendable for patients with renal disease for the lack of nephrotoxicity in the microbubbles [2]. Another feature of second-generation CM is the very low incidence of allergic reactions compared to gadolinium-based or iodinated CM. Currently, its use is indicated as unsafe in cases of: recent heart attack (<7 days), right to left shunt, severe pulmonary hypertension, pregnancy, lactation, or severe cardiac disease (III/IV class) [3]. In the execution of a contrast-enhanced ultrasound, one can make use of a wide range of software original to the apparatus. The current most frequently used technique is that referred to as conservative, or non-destructive: the acoustic pressure applied does not cause the microbubbles to burst, but uses non-linear oscillation to generate the echo amplification of the ultrasound signal. The pressure is measured by the mechanical index (MI). The conservative method uses a low MI, in contrast with the past use of the destructive method, in which the amplified ultrasound signal was achieved, after having broken the microbubbles, by employing a raised MI with the intensity of the signal with a shorter duration [2, 4].

G. Regine et al., *Contrast-Enhanced Ultrasound of the Urinary Tract*,
DOI: 10.1007/978-88-470-5432-5_1, © Springer-Verlag Italia 2013

1.2   Research Method

In line with other published studies, the research method of urinary tract pathology we have chosen consists of a baseline evaluation, then integrated with color Doppler, and followed by the contrast-enhanced phase: access to a peripheral vein is used, usually the antecubital vein of the arm, first administering an intravenous (IV) bolus of 1.2 mL of Sonovue (Bracco SpA, Milano, Italia), followed by 10 mL of saline solution, if necessary, in a second bolus. The ultrasound systems we used are of the Siemens Sequoia brand (Siemens Medical Solutions, USA Inc., Mountain View, CA), with Cadence Pulse Sequencing (CPS) technology and a low mechanical index (<0.2) [4]. Sonograms were acquired through image recording with Picture Archiving and Communication System (PACS) using real time imaging for a varying duration, depending on the organ, ranging from 2 to 5 min, with an early arterial phase (the moment in which the arrival of microbubbles in the vascular renal hilum is first noted and the 20 s following), a late arterial phase (up to around 40 s) and a late/parenchymal phase (up to 5 min) [1, 3]. The images can be recorded not only by enhancing the contrast effect (AC method), but also by using a blended method in which the software also provides a grayscale B-mode version of the image (Fig. 1.1). Contrast-enhanced ultrasound, therefore, is multi-phased like computed tomographic (CT) and magnetic resonance (MRI), but allows, once the microbubbles are destroyed by color Doppler signal (using, if necessary, a second bolus) a more targeted image of the lesion-affected organ, on which basis it should be considered a dynamic process [5, 6]. All of the cases documented in the present publication were integrated with one or even two other methods of imaging, specifically with a TC exam (Aquilion, 64 rows, Toshiba, Japan) using multi-phase integrated technique reconstructing 3D ultrasound

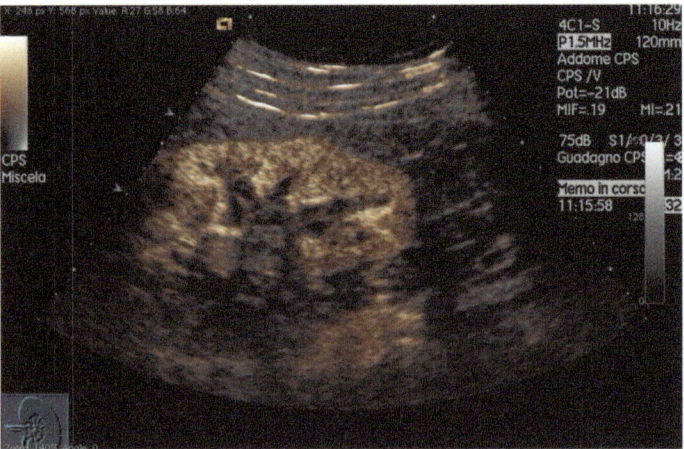

Fig. 1.1 Blended modality ultrasound exam: it is possible to see both the grayscale imaging, and the contrast effect of microbubbles

images; and/or with MRI exams (Signa 1.5 T, GE, USA) using the sequences T1, T2, T1 with fat suppression and 3D Spoiled Gradient. Clearly malignant lesions were referred to surgical treatment and subsequent histological evaluation; those images which gave suspicion were followed up with biopsy evaluation.

1.3   Terminology

The kidney, a richly vascularized organ, responds with a rapid and intense amplification of the sonographic signal in the early and late arterial phases throughout the parenchyma, with the exception of the bone marrow; and thereafter, in the late/parenchymal phase, we see a homogenous saturation of the entire renal parenchyma [5–7]. Parenchymal abnormalities, which appear as un-vascularized areas, can be detected in each of the phases of the exam (ischemia, infarcts, inflammation, traumatic lesions), with a fairly small margin of error, in triangular, linear or irregular shapes; also manifested as regions with a higher saturation during one or more phases of the exam, or a lower saturation in the arterial or late phase. These variations, if properly correlated, help not only in the identification but also in the characterization of the lesion [5–8]. For convenience, we have divided our experience into three types of application of ultrasound, each of which presents its own technical aspects and pathology:

(1) Renal
(2) Urinary tract and bladder
(3) Evaluation of vesicoureteral reflux.

References

1. Claudon M, Cosgrove D, Albrecht T et al (2008) Guidelines and good clinical practice recommendations for contrast enhanced ultrasound (CEUS), update 2008. Ultraschall Med 29:28–44
2. Quaia E (2007) Microbubble ultrasound contrast agents: an update. Eur Radiol 17:1995–2008
3. Prakash A, Tan GJ, Wansaicheong GK (2011) Contrast enhanced ultrasound of kidneys. Pictorial essay. Med Ultrason 13:150–156
4. Wilson SR, Burns PN (2010) Microbubble-enhanced US in body imaging: what role? Radiology 257:24–39
5. Siracusano S, Bertolotto M, Ciciliato S et al (2011) The current role of contrast-enhanced ultrasound (CEUS) imaging in the evaluation of renal pathology. World J Urol 29:633–638
6. Setola SV, Catalano O, Sandomenico F, Siani A (2007) Contrast-enhanced sonography of the kidney. Abdom Imaging 32:21–28
7. Siracusano S, Quaia E, Bertolotto M et al (2004) The application of ultrasound contrast agents in the characterization of renal tumors. World J Urol 22:316–322
8. Valentino M, Serra C, Zironi G et al (2006) Blunt abdominal trauma: emergency contrast-enhanced sonography for detection of solid organ injuries. AJR Am J Roentgenol 186:1361–1367

The Kidney

2

The applications of the use of second generation CM in the field of renal pathology includes the following types of diseases: ischemic, traumatic, inflammatory and expansive (the latter includes both cystic and solid masses). Another use is in cases of kidney transplants, in which software is now available to give a quantitative analysis that can define levels of parenchymal perfusion and determine the Intensity/Time curves.

2.1 Ischemic Pathology

The use of ultrasound in the evaluation of renal ischemia provides a level of diagnostic accuracy comparable to that of CT. Documented experience of various Authors confirms that the diagnostic performance of the method is high and the comparative advantage is in the elimination of the need to use contract media that are potentially nephrotoxic for patients who, because of specific health conditions, may have already reduced kidney functionality (calculated on the basis of the glomular filtration rate), in addition to not using ionizing radiation [1–3]. After the infusion of the CM, the ischemic area is visible as a well-defined region with does not show post-sonographic enhancement in the various phases of the exam. The high-quality spatial resolution also makes it possible to differentiate between renal infarction and cortical ischemia, which is characterized by the saturation of the segmentary, interlobar, or arcuate vascular structures, which cannot be detected at the level of the interlobular vessels of the renal cortex [1–5]. Our observations confirm other published findings: in a series of 16 patients with ischemic regions identified in a previous multi-slice CT scan (MSCT), in 13 cases we obtained an image comparable to the reference scan on the second day, although in the 3

G. Regine et al., *Contrast-Enhanced Ultrasound of the Urinary Tract*,
DOI: 10.1007/978-88-470-5432-5_2, © Springer-Verlag Italia 2013

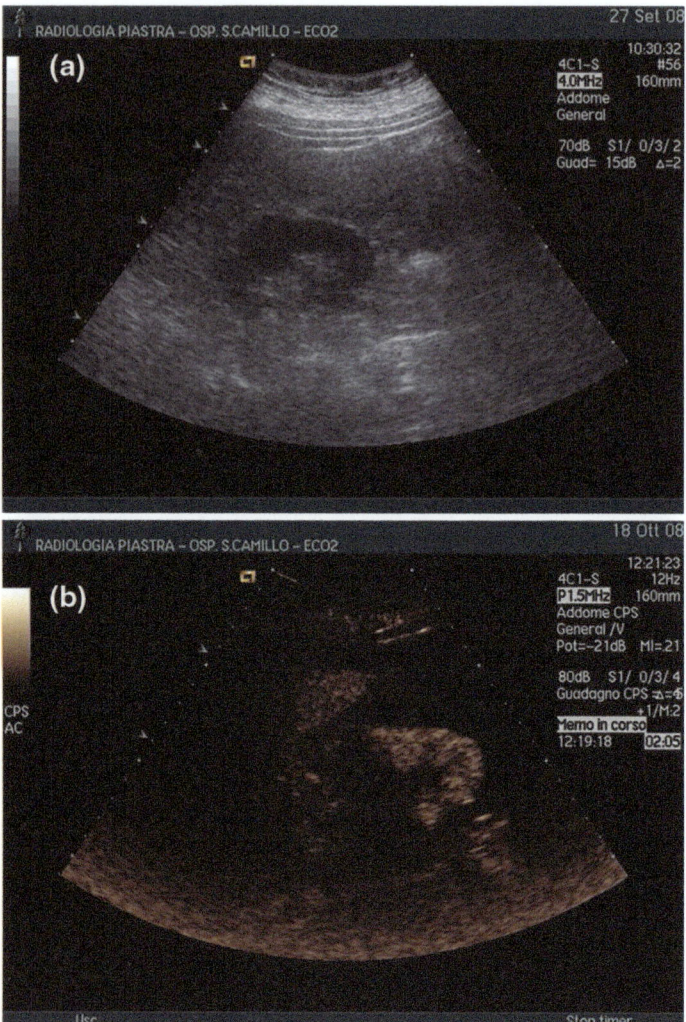

Fig. 2.1 Baseline exam that appears negative; late CEUS image in the late phase shows a triangular avascular area with a cortical base with ischemic traits (**a**, **b**). **c** The cortico-medullary phase of the MSCT scan highlights a finding that fully matches that of the CEUS exam

remaining cases the onset and/or aggravation of cardiocirculatory problems made it impossible to perform the test. This observation caused us to follow up our findings with these patients using only sonographic tests until its resolution, and this was confirmed by an evaluation using MSCT which showed a perfect overlap between the two imaging techniques. This was the case in 8 of the 13 patients monitored; in the remaining 5, due to the persistence of ischemic regions and associated parenchymal retraction, follow-up was done using CEUS alone (Fig. 2.1).

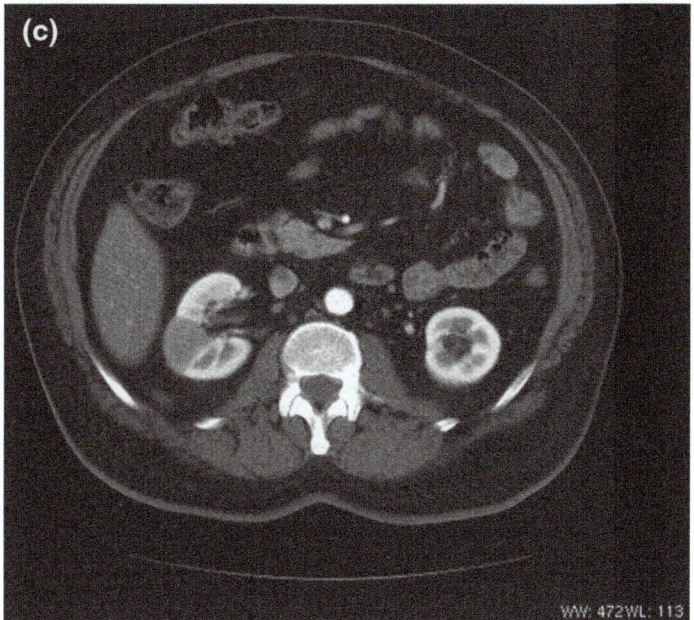

Fig. 2.1 (continued)

2.2 Traumatic Pathology

In order to speak about trauma, it becomes necessary to define the term. In the most severe cases of trauma, CEUS would not be the first choice among procedures: this type of patient must be evaluated using MSCT, a technique with the advantages of a high spatial and temporal resolution, coverage of wide corporal bodies, the narrowness of the slice, quick execution time and the possibility to build 2D and 3D reconstructions [6, 7].

Contrast-enhances ultrasound is recommended in minor traumas or more severe traumas in stable patients, or to follow up on renal lesions which appear on the MSCT scan. Both from the review of literature [6, 8] and on the basis of our case studies, we find CEUS is a quick and simple means to identify various types of renal lesions: lacerations appear as avascular regions with fairly ragged borders which extends in an irregular way across the healthy parenchyma (Fig. 2.2); in severe cases it is impossible to recognize the normal renal appearance. The peri- and parirenal hematoma is visible, with possible signs of active bleeding, often associated with lacerations, indicated by a blush of contract medium, which can be seen in the early phase of the exam (Fig. 2.3). The vascular renal hilum lesion is characterized by a complete lack of post-ultrasound saturation of the parenchyma. This occurrence, like renal lesions of a high degree, are difficult to notice using CEUS, inasmuch as they usually are found in poly-traumatized and or unstable patients [7].

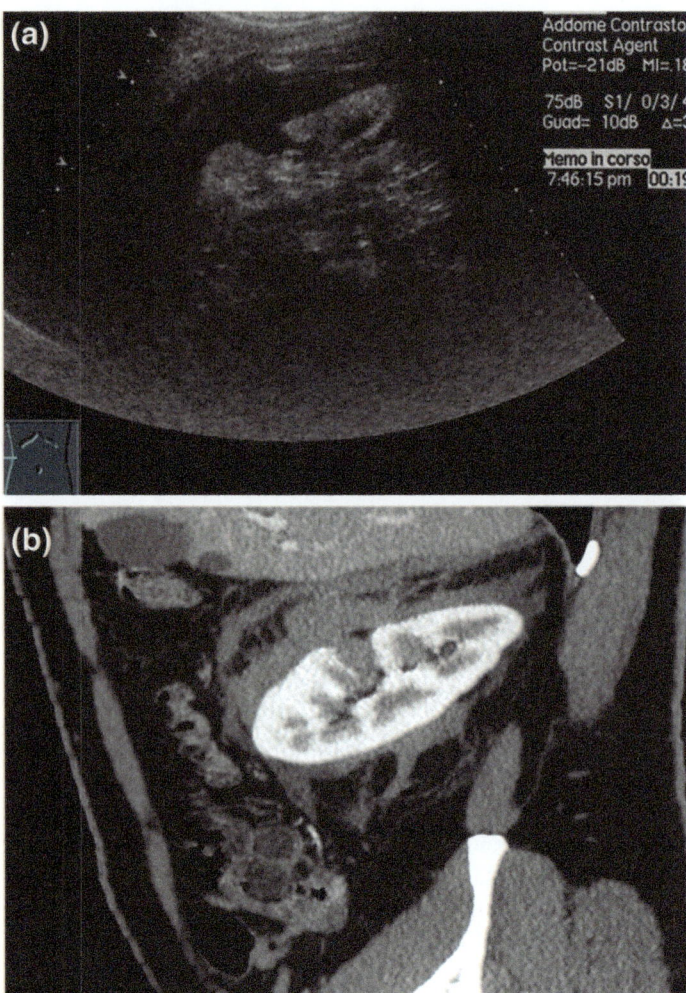

Fig. 2.2 **a** Laceration of the upper pole of the right kidney: CEUS shows a thin linear avascular area with perirenal hematoma. **b** MSCT scan, after intravenous infusion of contrast agent, displays the same as (**a**), with substantially similar results

In our experience over the course of 2 years, we have evaluated 255 stable patients with minor closed trauma, with and without hematuria; and using CEUS we have identified 28 lesions confirmed by MSCT, and by comparison of the images distinguished three levels of damage: minor (corresponds more or less with grade 1 of the American Association for the Surgery of Trauma—AAST), medium (corresponds with grades 2 and 3 of AAST classification) and high (corresponds with grade 3 and 4 of AAST classification) [7]. Experience has also shown that in cases of minor trauma, with ribs lesions, of "parasurgical" operations on the kidney

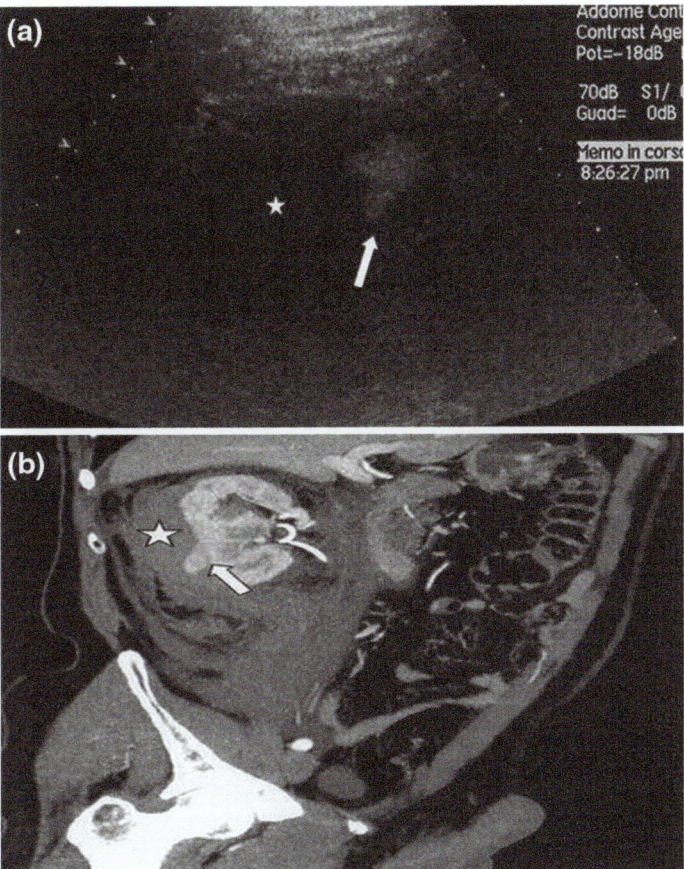

Fig. 2.3 **a** Static image, extrapolated by dynamic recording in video clips, displays both extensive pararenal bruising (*star*), and an active exstavasation (*blush*) of the ultrasound contrast agent (*arrow*) indicating a lesion of the renal cortical vessels after lithotripsy. **b** MSCT scan (multi-planar reconstruction) of the case of (**a**) which identifies the same highlighted findings of the CEUS exam: pararenal hematoma (*star*) and blush (*arrow*)

(lithotripsy, biopsy, nephrostomy, etc.) with hematuria, rapid and progressive anemia, the baseline ultrasound should always be supplemented by a CEUS evaluation. The main limit of the method is found in the lack of a means to evaluate the integrity of the urinary tract in relationship with the lack of excretion with that means of CM. Another application is for follow-up: considering the diagnostic overlapping of CEUS with MSTC, it is mandatory, on the bases both of our case studies as well as current literature [1, 6–8], to carry out the monitoring of the evolution of traumatic renal lesions using CEUS, in order to achieve the following goals: to avoid use of radiation for patients (often young ones), to avoid the use of nephrotoxic agents, more adequate diagnostic accuracy and cost savings.

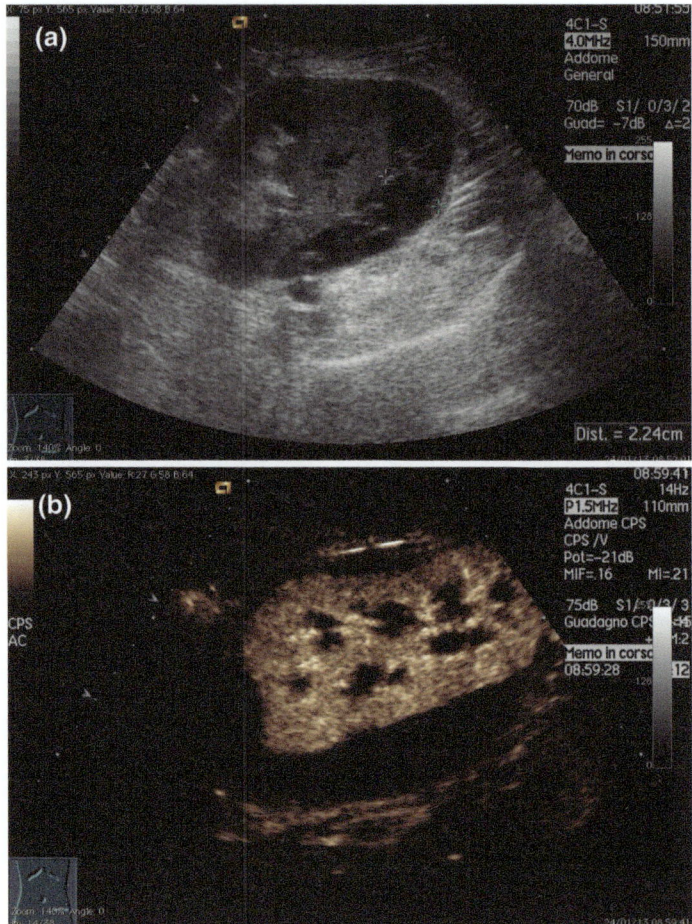

Fig. 2.4 Perirenal fluid collection: the baseline (**a**) does not permit the definition of the extension and nature. The CEUS image (**b–c**) identifies not only the extension and the homogeneously non-echogenic and non-corpuscular nature of the collection, compatible with seroma, but also shows the conditions of the parenchyma

2.3   Transplantation

CEUS is a non-invasive method which is useful in the identification of vascular and non-vascular complications in kidney transplant [1, 3, 5, 9]. Post-transplant complications can be early or late. Early complications arrive in the first week after

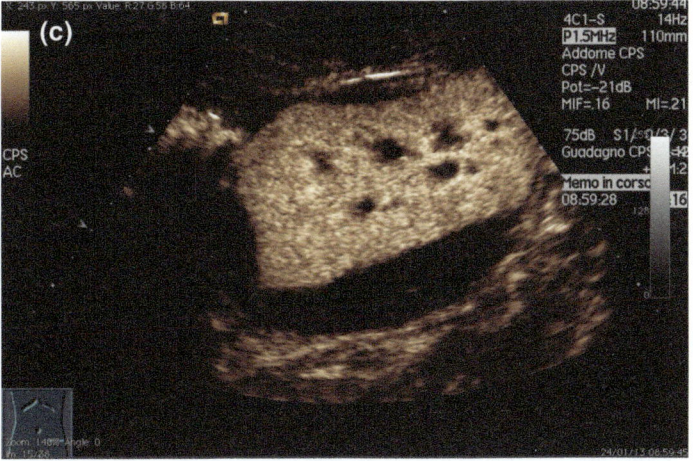

Fig. 2.4 (continued)

the transplant and include: acute rejection, tubular necrosis, hematoma, pyelone-phritis, abscess, urinoma, ureteral obstructions, or vascular obstructions [10, 11]. Late complications appear beginning several weeks after the transplant and include: chronic rejection, ureteral obstructions, cysts, cancer, and complications related to immunosuppressive therapies, such as for lymphoma and cancer, and infections particularly risky in kidney transfer [10–13]. In adults, the transplanted kidney is placed in the heterotopic extraperitoneale space in the iliac fossa with end-to-side anastomosis between the renal artery and the external or common iliac artery. The vesicoureteral anastomosis is usually done close to the trigone, with the creation of a submucous tunnel that prevents reflux.

2.3.1 Perirenal and Renal Fluid Collections

These are frequent and include hematoma, (late) lymphocele, (early) seroma, abscess, and urinoma. In CEUS these collections appear with no enhancement: using this procedure it is possible to define them and establish the anatomic relationships with adjacent structures (Fig. 2.4a–c). Additionally, the method can be of help in cases of puncture and drainage.

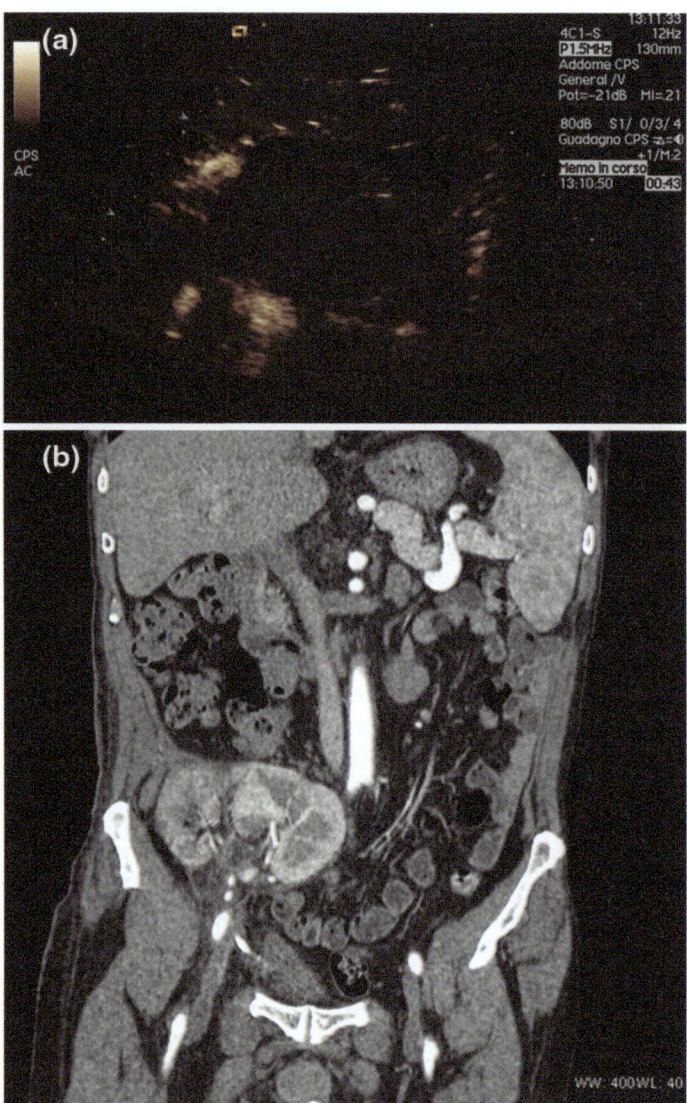

Fig. 2.5 a Transplanted kidney with stenosis of the arterial iliac-renal anastomosis: the CEUS shows a widespread reduction in parenchymal perfusion. **b** MSCT (coronal reconstruction) confirms the presence of an area of reduced saturation after the infusion of contrast medium

2.3.2   Vascular Complications

Renal and iliac artery stenosis

The first is usually found in the perianastomotic zone, is the most common vascular complication and can be found at both early and late stages. Stenotic

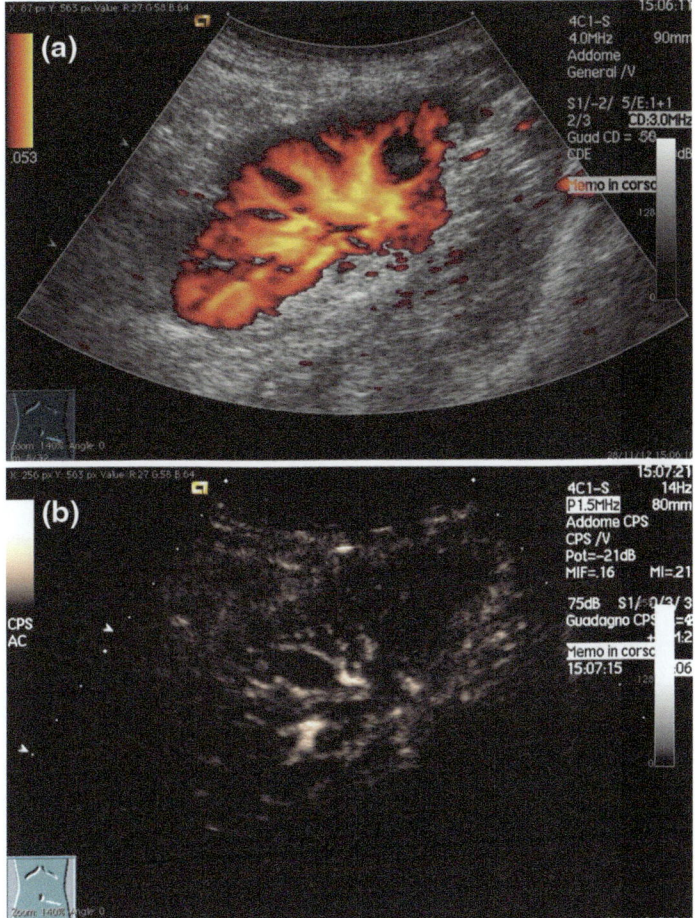

Fig. 2.6 **a–d** Sectoral lack of vascularization in the lower polar region of the transplanted kidney, evaluated with the Power-Doppler (**a**). Multi-phase CEUS confirms the area with no perfusion indicative of hypoperfusion, which appears to be extended beyond (**b–c**)

complications are due to the onset of arterial hypertension after the transplant. In the case of hemodynamically significant stenosis, CEUS shows perfusion defects in the renal parenchyma that can affect the entire parenchyma (Fig. 2.5) or only select regions, most often peripheral ones, such as the polar regions bordering both ischemic regions and hypoperfused neighboring zones (Fig. 2.6). [1, 9, 11, 14]

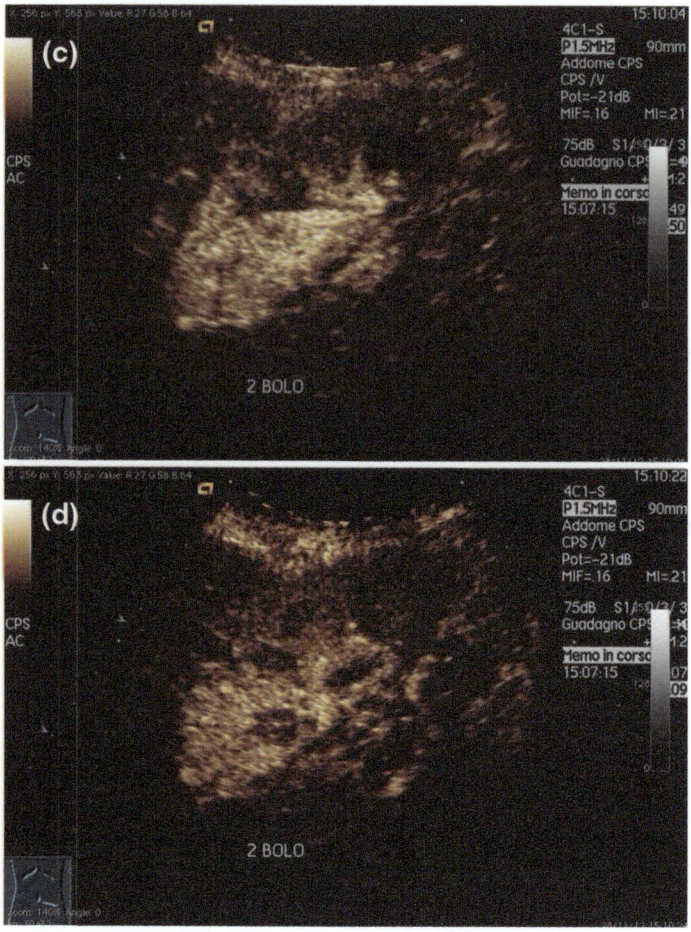

Fig. 2.6 (continued)

Renal artery thrombosis

Thrombosis of the renal artery is a vascular complication with immediate systemic or surgical causes. It causes renal infarctions due to lack of parenchymal enhancement and capsular enhancement [1, 10, 15].

Intrarenal pseudoaneurysms and arteriovenous fistulas

These are iatrogenic complications that follow a percutaneous biopsy. The first are subsequent to an arteriovenous laceration, the second after an exclusively arterial lesion [11–13]. In our experience, we found that the presence of a stenosis of the

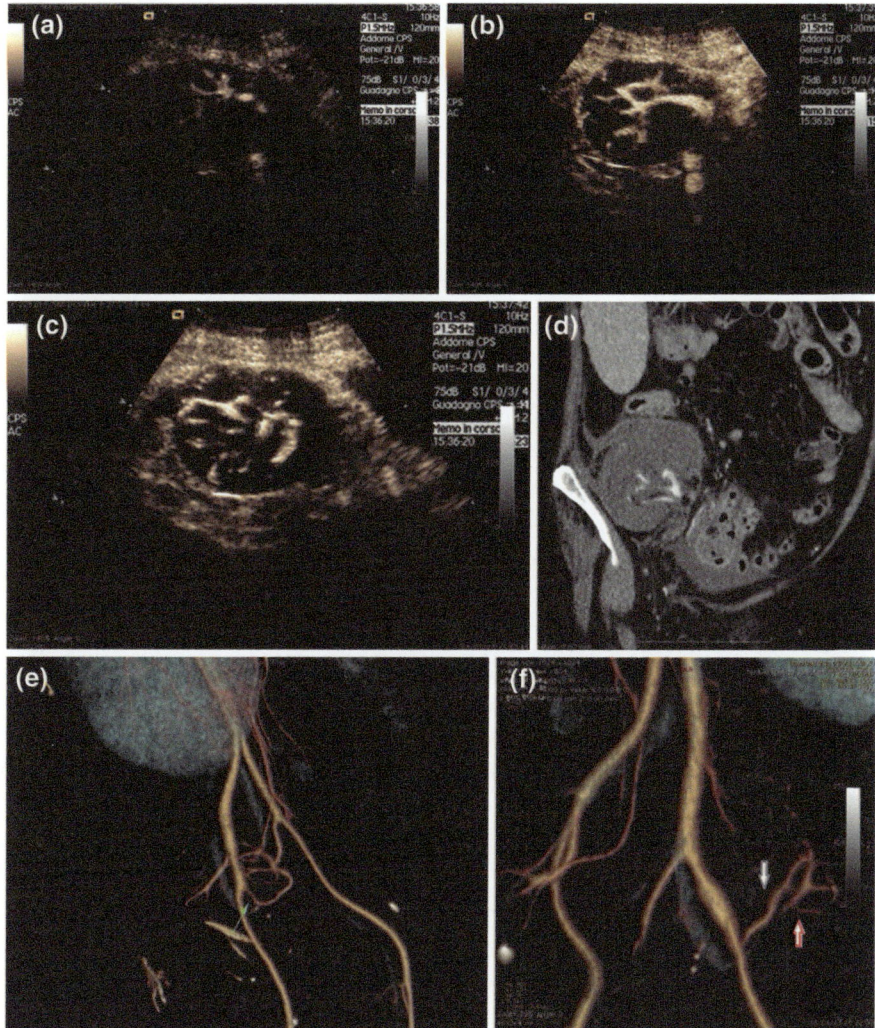

Fig. 2.7 **a–f** Integrated CEUS and MSCT imaging of renal artery stenosis anastomosed with the external iliac artery (*arrow*) and (**e**) and a post-biopsy fistula in an acute rejection with simultaneous opacity of the artery (**f**) (*gray arrow*) and renal vein (*red arrow*). The more panoramic view of MSCT allows for a diagnosis; CEUS identified the absence of parenchymal perfusion and heavy saturation of the two vascular compartments (**a–c**)

renal artery, anastomosed with the iliac artery, was linked to the presence of an arteriovenous fistula that developed after a biopsy to assess a rejection, which in the case study was indicated by the absence of perfusion (Fig. 2.7).

Extrarenal pseudoaneurysms

Usually asymptomatic, these are related to surgical technique and are rarely infectious.

Renal artery thrombosis

Early complication due to incorrect surgical technique or systemic causes, or late complication due to chronic rejection. It is possible to see the thrombus and persistent nephrographic effect in the late phase.

Renal artery stenosis

Stenosis in the renal artery is rare and is caused by incorrect surgical technique or perirenal alterations such as fibrosis or extrinsic compression from perirenal masses [12, 13].

2.3.3 Urological Complications

Urinoma

Complication secondary to ureteral extravasation following rejection, ischemic ureteral necrosis or incorrect surgical technique. CT Urography or RM Urography can show any ureteral leak and the passage of the CM in the collection. CEUS picks up the collection as a mass with no enhancement, but does not identify the seat of the extravasation, as there is no pyelographic phase [12, 13, 15].

Ureteral strictures

In these cases, CEUS has no role. May be evaluated using uroCT scan or uroMRI.

Acute and chronic rejections

Acute rejection and acute tubular necrosis are the most frequent causes of unsuccessful transplants. Signaled by appearance of an alteration in the cortico-medullary differentiation and a reduced nephrographic effect after the CEUS. Chronic rejection is caused by sclerosant vasculitis and by interstitial fibrosis, which leads to reduced renal profusion [12, 16]. For transplant patients, CEUS is a quick, non-invasive and repeatable method with no negative side effect on renal functionality. A blood pool contrast medium is used, which displays the state of parenchymal perfusion in cases of suspected vascular complications or rejection, integrating the findings with color Doppler. Useful in the location and monitoring of collections, it does not provide information for urological complications as it does not include the excretion phase [5, 15].

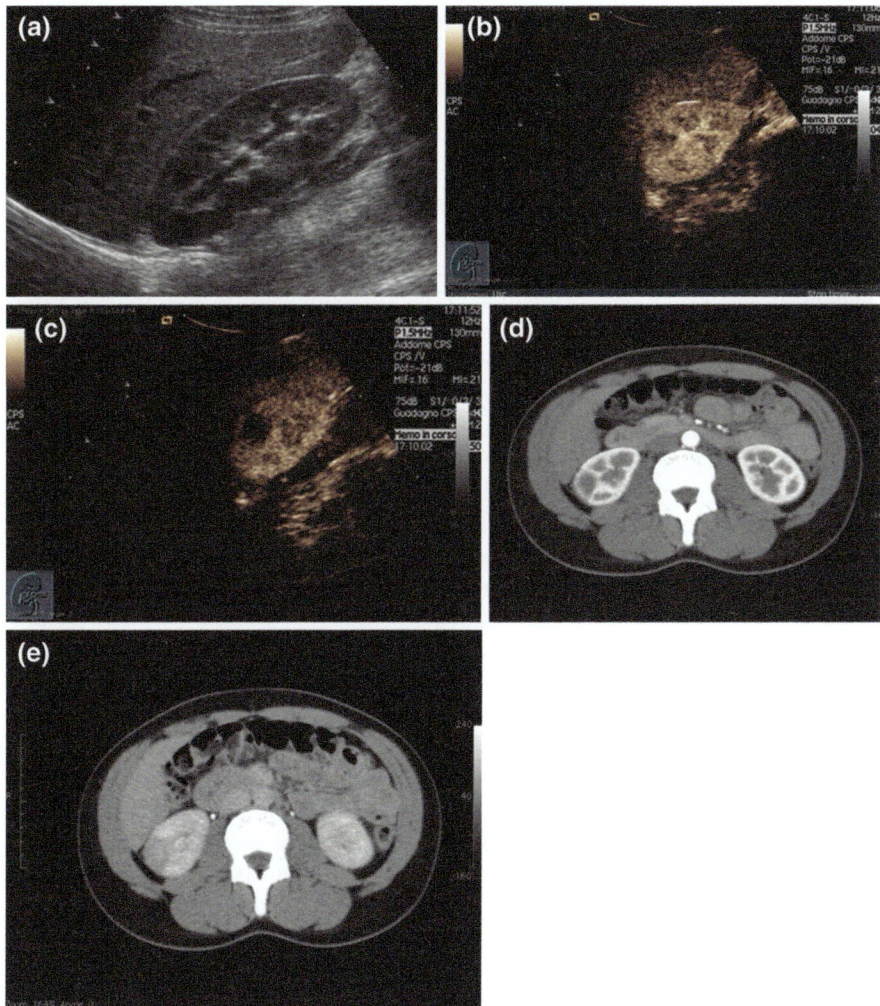

Fig. 2.8   **a–e** Baseline examination in patients with inflammation of the urinary tract which shows no abnormalities; **b–c**: CEUS image in the late arterial phase with parenchyma showing signs of a cortico-subcortical avascular area, most defined in the late phase (**c**) **d–e**: Multiphase CT scan with concordant findings

2.4   Inflammation Pathology

For inflammations, the consultation of imaging is often used in cases of a suspected or known complication, either local or systemic, in order to clarify the nature and the extension, and when possible, to identify the cause [17].

The imaging technique of choice is MSCT with the intravenous (IV) infusion of the CM, but increasing observations in current literature confirm that CEUS has equal diagnostic accuracy, with the advantages of no ionizing radiation exposure and the use of a non-nephrotoxic CM [1, 5, 9, 17, 18]. We will not dwell on the clinical-laboratory accumulated data on renal inflammation, the consideration of which is of course a fundamental element of diagnosis, but rather we seek to define the role of CEUS in the differential diagnosis between focal pyelonephritis and abscess and between focal pyelonephritis and an ischemic zone, monitoring the possible outcomes. This is essential to properly manage the treatment of the patient. In our experience (19 patients), focal pyelonephritis appeared as a hypo-echoic, and not vascularized, area with cortical or corticomedullary localization which appeared in a more defined way in the parenchymal phase (Fig. 2.8). Aligning with current literature [4, 17, 18], the findings described are often variable and often a negative analysis can come with the help of a comparison with the two preceding phases. In fact, in 16 out of 19 patients with suspected focal pyelonephritis, the lesion appeared hypoechoic in the arterial phase, and then became isoechoic to the parenchyma in the late arterial phase, and finally in the late parenchymal phase turned again to be hypoechoic. In 5 of the 13 patients, round areas with avascular characteristics could be seen in these triangular-shaped hypoechoic zones. Some of these showed peripheral saturation which resembled an abscess (Fig. 2.9). In the remaining 3 patients, the sonogram primarily displayed one or more abscess lesions accompanied by cortical bulging and a fluid perirenal reaction. Results of follow-up showed that in all forms of pyelonephritis without microabscesses, there was a complete resolution; accordingly, in cases with the presence of abscesses we observed a parenchymal retraction with contextual evidence of a fibrotic scar and sectorial regions of parenchymal atrophy. Let us recall that this method can be used for the differential diagnostic between pyelonephritis and focal ischemia, as was already mentioned in the paragraph on infarctic lesions. It seems from this that a more wide-spread use of this methodology is to be encouraged in the study of inflammation pathology, integrating it in cases of clinical doubt with baseline examinations using IV contrast medium in order to enhance the diagnostic accuracy, which otherwise remains markedly inferior to that of MSTC. This conclusion is reinforced by the advantages described at the beginning of this paragraph and by the possibility of simultaneous identification of possible triggers (urolithiasis).

2.5   Solid Lesions

Numerous published studies [19–21] have evaluated the diagnostic trustworthiness of the technique, not only in finding of lesions, but also in their characterization. Currently, it seems certain that the use of CEUS is mandatory in cases in which B-mode scans have been inconclusive and/or nullifying, as the integration of the two techniques considerably increases the diagnostic accuracy [5, 9]. Once the lesion has been identified, the next step is, as has been stated, is its

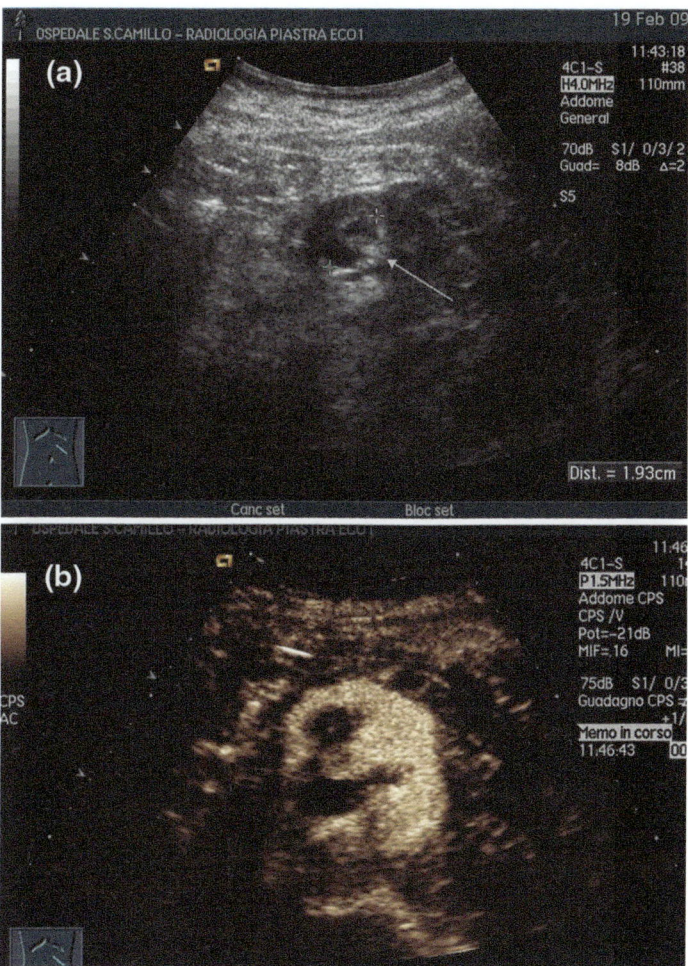

Fig. 2.9 Evaluation of an abscess formation in the parapyelic space of the left kidney. Baseline examination (**a**), arterial phase (**b**), late parenchymal phase (**c**) delimitation of abscess formation, suspected in the baseline, and the late phase CEUS image also detects an area of peripheral saturation (*arrow*). **d** Same case evaluated by MSCT: delimitation of the abscess capsule (*arrow*)

characterization. This is a fundamental question, considering that in recent years, both because of an increase in the availability of effective equipment and because of a higher propensity to perform routine examinations, one is faced with increasing the number of subjects with renal lesions, often small and difficult to classify. Resulting from this is an increased demand for surgery, even for injuries that are not always histologically found malignant.

One must remember that, from the histological point of view, solid kidney lesions can be either benign or malignant. Renal carcinomas fall under several histological subtypes: among the most frequent are clear cells (70–80 %), then

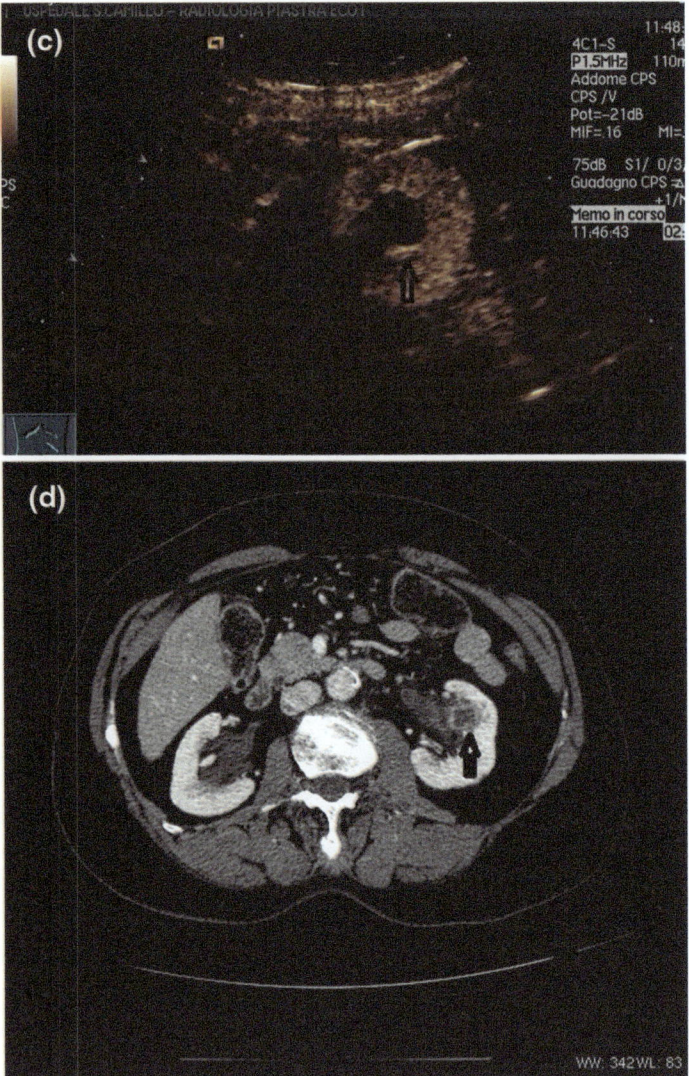

Fig. 2.9 (continued)

papillary cells (10–15 %), chromophobe cells (5 %), and medullary carcinoma and collecting ducts (1–2 %). Among the benign lesions are angiomiolipona and oncocytoma, which is sometimes to be considered as a borderline lesion. The various forms have differing macroscopic features (necrotic, hemorrhaging, cystic degeneration); while from the microscopic point of view we can see varying levels of cellularity that influence the vascular component. Another aspect to consider is that of growth patterns, which can be considered expansive especially in the clear, papillary and chromophobe form, but is infiltrative in carcinoma of the collection

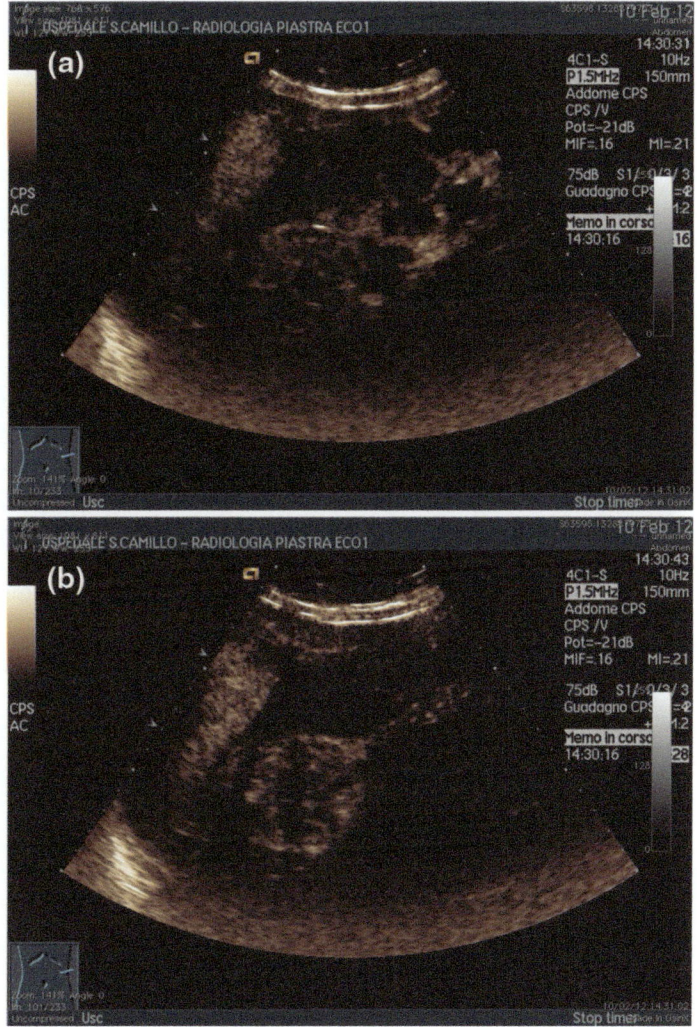

Fig. 2.10   a–c CEUS appearance of a clear cell lesion of the upper pole of the left kidney: note the late-stage detection of a pseudocapsule (*arrows*). **d** Corresponding MSCT scan: coronal reconstruction in parenchymal phase

ducts and bone marrow [22]. Another aspect of characterization is determined by the presence of a pseudocapsule, typical sign of an expansive pattern, which consists of peripheral fibrous tissue, secondary to the development of ischemic phenomena and of necrosis in healthy tissue adjacent to the lesion [23]. The various authors who have used the methodology in the evaluation of renal masses, despite presenting case studies which are numerically variable [19, 20, 24, 25], are in agreement concerting the definition of sufficient semiological aspects to provide an aid in the characterization of lesions based on their distinct histologic traits: the

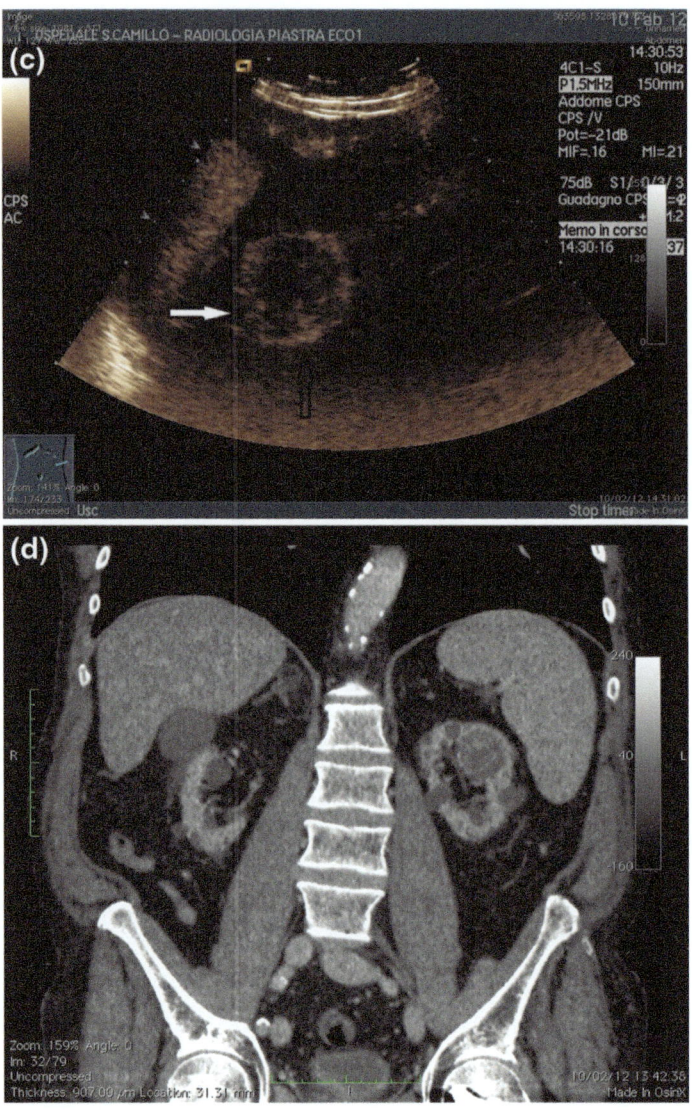

Fig. 2.10 (continued)

degree of vascularization, magnitude of the washout and, lastly, the presence or absence of pseudocapsule. The clear cell forms, according to the majority of the authors cited, demonstrate an uneven enhancement in the early arterial phase, which at times appears relatively less intense than the surrounding healthy parenchyma; in the late arterial phase the lesion becomes more homogeneous due to washout, then in the late phase they tend to become more echogenic, but with a richly vascularized peripheral capsule called a pseudocapsule (Fig. 2.10).

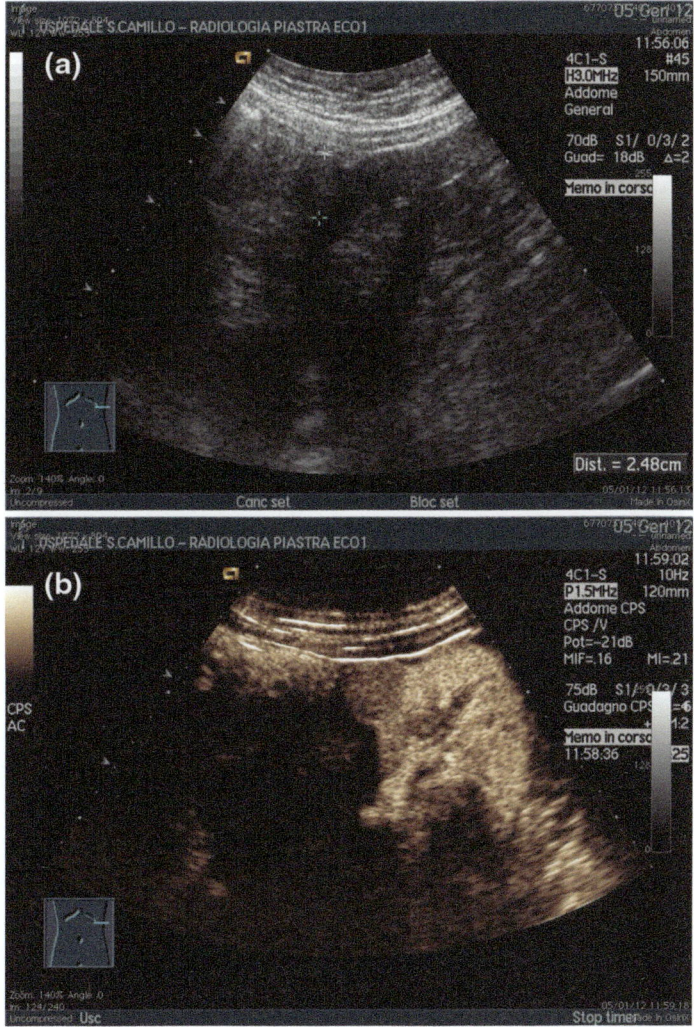

Fig. 2.11 a–d Polar injury to top of the left kidney. Examination at baseline: nodular cortical area. The CEUS displays low post-contrast enhancement both in the arterial (**b**) and late (**c**) phases; as well as the post- contrast MSCT scan (**d**). Histological evaluation gave a diagnosis of a papillary form

The papillary cell forms have a minimal, but in any case uneven, post-contrast enhancement in the late arterial phase, with subsequent continuous and constant washout in the following stages; and the mass tends to become more hypoechoic compared to the healthy surrounding parenchyma, with the possible identification of a pseudocapsule (Fig. 2.11) [21, 25, 26].

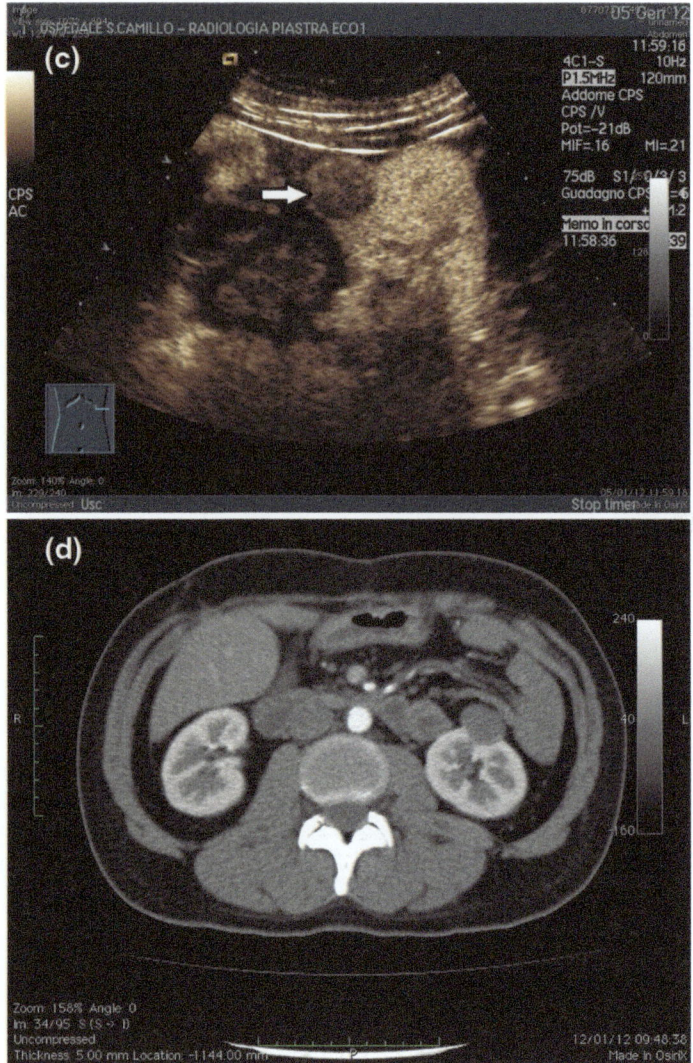

Fig. 2.11 (continued)

Angiomyolipoma, according to various authors, appears in CEUS with a homogeneous and prolonged post-contrast enhancement (Fig. 2.12), although it often does not manifest a certain pattern and the CEUS appears to be at a disadvantage compared to other imaging techniques [19, 26, 27]. In fact, in our

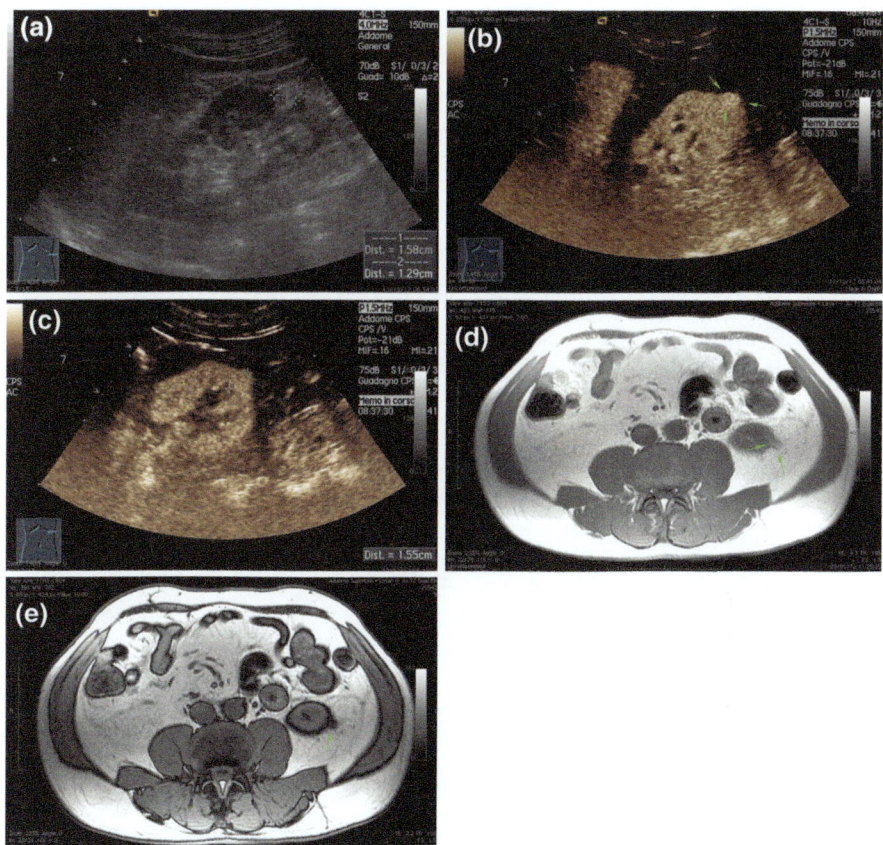

Fig. 2.12 Evaluation with baseline examination (**a**) early phase CEUS (**b**) and parenchymal phase (**c**), and MRI with sequences in phase and in phase opposition (**d–e**). The hyperechoic formation during baseline phase shows persistent and homogeneous saturation in both phases. Confirmation of the finding of a fat containing formation with MRI

experience we found ourselves in doubtful cases where the post-contrast behavior was ambiguous, which can sometimes create diagnostic problems which can most be attributed to the varying components that make up the formation (Fig. 2.13).

Oncocytoma is the second most common benign neoplasm after angiomyolipoma. In CEUS evaluations, it can be recognized by the presence in the early arterial phase of a wagon wheel shape, and subsequent homogenous enhancement of the lesion in the late arterial phase; in the parenchymal phase it becomes isoechoic with a central hypoechoic scar (Fig. 2.14) [21]. The oncocytoma does

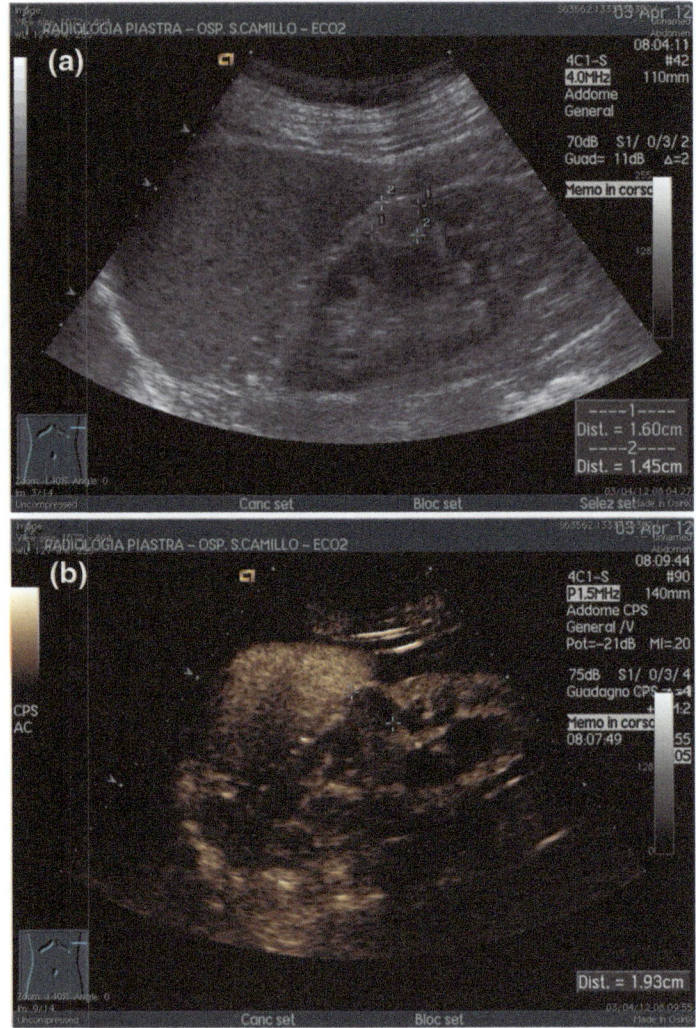

Fig. 2.13 Angiomio-lipomatosic formation in the left kidney that appears tenuously hyperechoic in baseline examination (**a**), with sonographic pattern characterized by an absent and/or reduced post-contrast saturation (**b**), while the MSCT in direct phase (**c**) and post-contrast enhancement (**d**) identifies and defines the nature of the lesion. This case demonstrates the poor ability of the methodology in characterization of angiomiolipoma

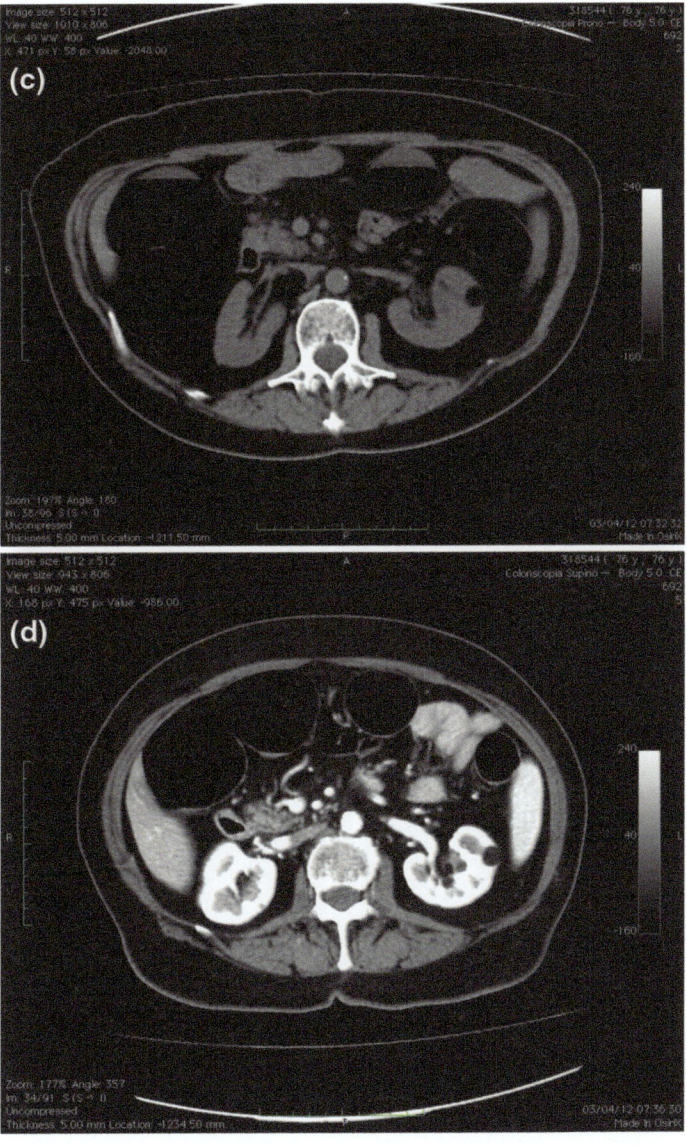

Fig. 2.13 (continued)

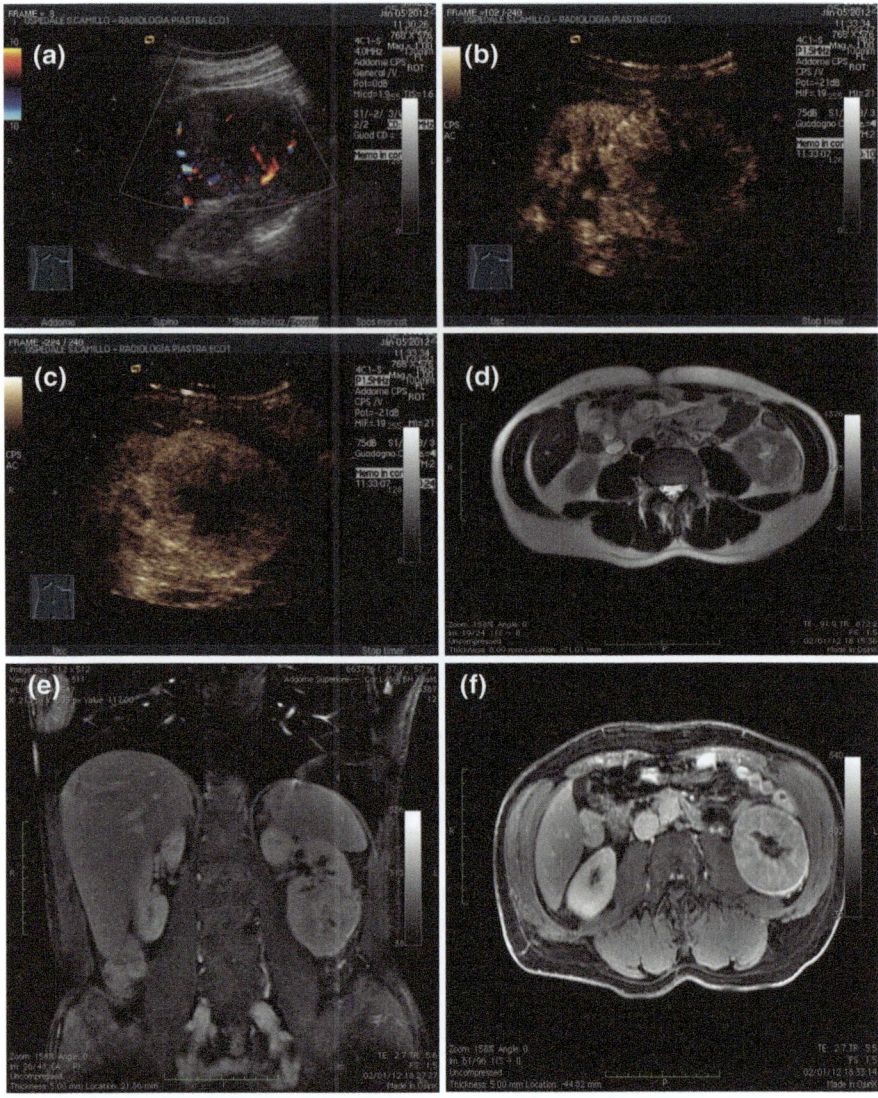

Fig. 2.14 Voluminous oncocytoma on the lower pole of the left kidney, evaluated with echo color Doppler system (**a**), with CEUS (**b, c**), and with MRI (**d–f**) with T2 and T1 with fat suppression sequences, according to axial and coronal planes after the IV infusion of contrast medium → paramagnetic. Both contrast techniques are able to highlight the pathognomonic aspects of the lesion (wheel-like appearance and central scar) giving comparable results

not always, however, have a central scar; it is often absent, or of such small dimensions and that it is barely noticeable (Fig. 2.15). At other times it is accompanied by the presence of a pseudocapsule of an intense and peritumoral vascularity that can be seen in the late phase (Fig. 2.16). These are the most typical

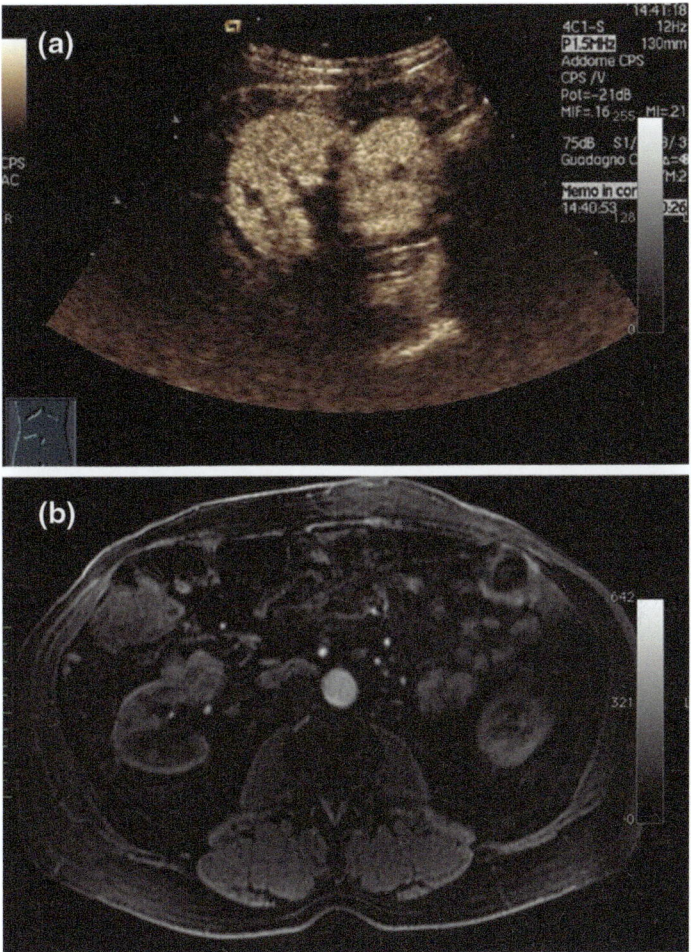

Fig. 2.15 **a–b** Expansive formation on the right kidney assessed by CEUS exam (**a**) and with MRI; the findings in both techniques appear nonspecific; there seems to be a thin scar in the central space, better defined on CEUS. Characterization obtained by biopsy showed it to be oncocytoma

aspects of the RCC, and so at times one must be very careful in differentiating the classic starry central scar of oncocytoma from the necrotic-colliquative region typical of adenocarcinoma. Sometimes the central star-shaped scar may appear hypervascular in the arterial phase; it also seems that the appearance of the scar is more constant in larger lesions [21] (Fig. 2.17a–e).

According to many authors, in general in the differential diagnosis of solid lesions, at least presumptively, and including possibly malignant and possibly benign forms, we must consider the following traits: the size and the grade and nature of post-contrast enhancement. The dimensions appear to directly affect the other two

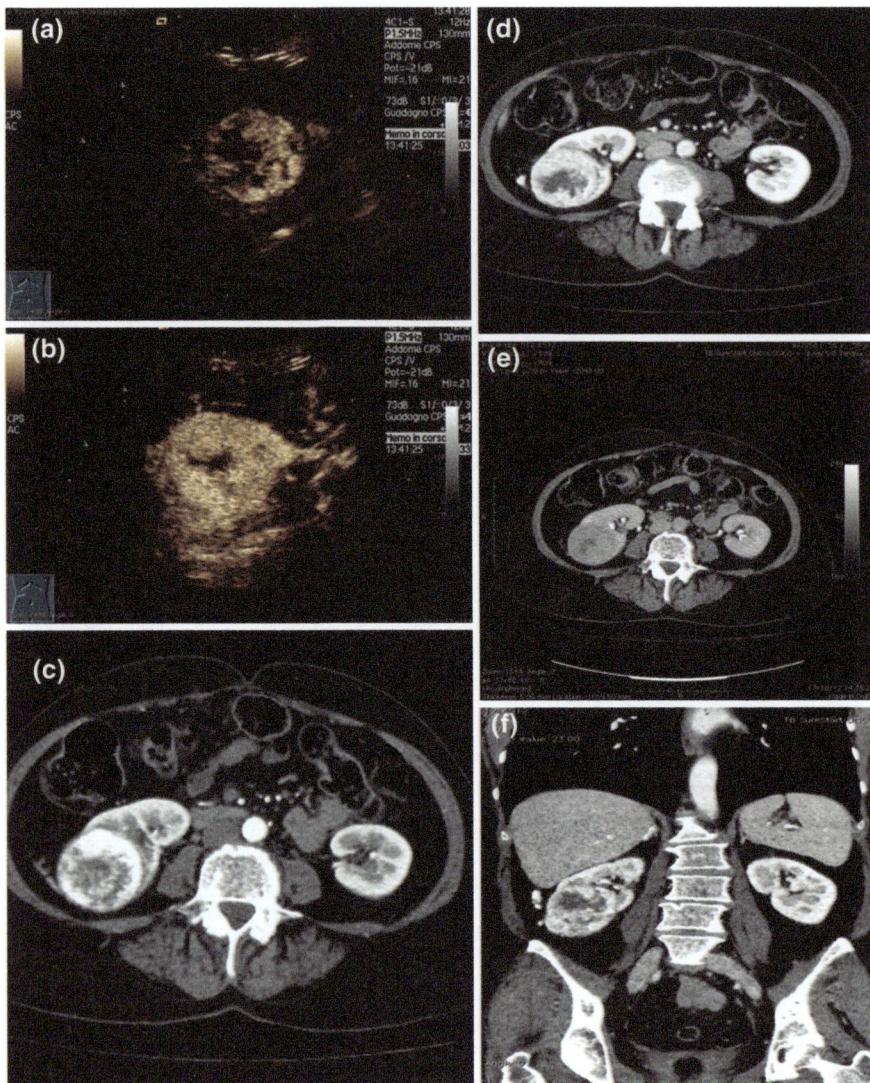

Fig. 2.16 Expansive formation assessed with contrast-enhanced ultrasound (**a–b**) and multi-phase CT scan (**c–d–e**), complemented by reconstructions according to the coronal plane (**f**) showing clinical findings typical of oncocytoma

aspects; insofar as large lesions are characterized by considerable unevenness in saturation with comparison to similar necrotic-colliquative intralesion phenomena. Another factor to take into consideration is the presence of a pseudocapsule, which as has been said, is better defined in the parenchymal phase and is almost always present in expansive formations with dimensions ranging between 2 and 5 cm [25, 27].

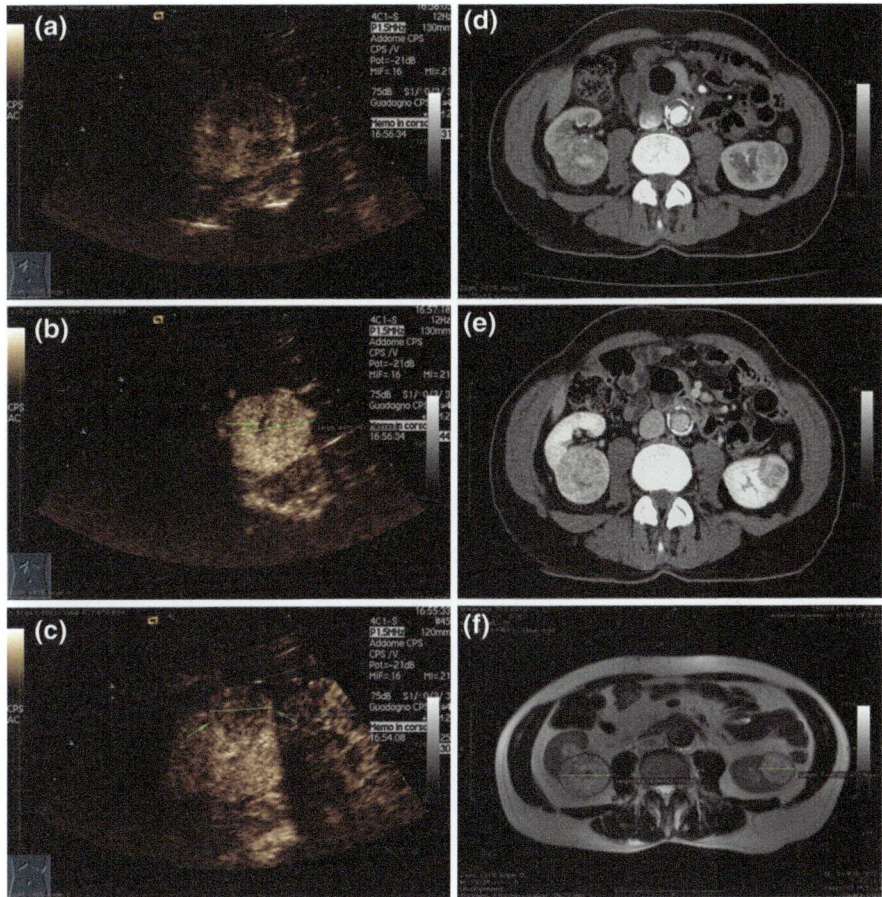

Fig. 2.17 **a–e** Evaluation with integrated imaging of bilateral oncocytoma. The lesion of the right kidney, which is larger, appears in the arterial CEUS phase (**a**) a hypervascular scar that tends in the late phase to be hypoechoic. Evaluation with CT and MRI (**d–e**)

In principle, invoking a concept valid for liver lesions, the presence of a wash-in early on, which persists in the arterial phase and appears non-homogeneous, with subsequent wash-out in the parenchymal phase and the possible development of a pseudocapsule, steers us towards a likely malignant lesion.

Conversely, the discovery of a continued contrastographic effect in the microbubbles within the lesion into the late phase, founds the argument for a possibly benign lesion.

Many authors [20, 28–31] have integrated the qualitative and quantitative aspects; with dedicated software it is possible to automatically compare the peak intensity and then create time/intensity curves at several locations of the renal parenchyma, thereby comparing the differences in behavior between healthy renal parenchyma and the site of an expansive lesion. It has been noted that the clear-cell malignancies demonstrate a lesser peak intensity in the early arterial phase compared to that of healthy renal parenchyma [20]. In reality, there exists in the literature a great variety of discordant observations with regard to the possibility of using CEUS for the characterization of a renal lesion, because such aspects as the size, the degree of necrosis and/or of hyalinization of the mass may hinder any attempt to use the technique [22, 24].

Our experience—consisting of a series of 47 patients evaluated in the period from November 2010 to December 2011—also revealed an objective difficulty in characterization of lesions; while there were no problems related to their detection.

The lesions identified using CEUS were classified, in terms of behavior, in forms with a high possibility of malignancy (rapid enhancement similar to that of the kidney in the early and late arterial phase, with subsequent washout which was slower than in renal cases, with uneven enhancement); and with an intermediate or low chance of malignancy (less intense enhancement than that of the kidney in all stages of the exam, with faster washout than in renal cases, fairly homogeneous enhancement, but occasional detection of nodular elements).

On the basis of this, have been identified 34/47 lesions with a potentially high degree of malignancy, 9/47 lesions with low-grade malignancy and 4/47 lesions that appear benign. All patients were evaluated with a second imaging technique (MSCT/MRI), with confirmation of the benignness of the four identified and characterized with CEUS (1 pseudo lesion, 3 angiomyolipomas); in 42 cases, indicative signs were confirmed by surgical excision approach, with the identification of metastatic lesions of lymphoma in the right kidney.

The surgical and histological assessments identified 29/42 clear cell tumors, 8/42 papillary cell tumors and 5/42 chromophobe cell tumors. Our study, not integrated with quantitative evaluation in all cases, is therefore limited considering that, according to some authors [20, 27, 28] it is from the integration of qualitative with quantitative data that it is possible to achieve a diagnostic accuracy in distinguishing the most potentially aggressive forms, and thereby set an appropriate plan of treatment.

Still, we would like to underline that our study has identified all lesions with the confirmation of secondary imaging and/or surgical methods, has correctly characterized benign lesions, while only slightly overestimating the percentage of those with a high grade of malignancy (72 vs. 69 %) in contrast with those with the lowest degree of malignancy.

The arrival of new software for quantitative analysis may help in the future to better define the behavior of lesions, and thereby to more accurately determine the degree of aggressiveness.

2.6   Cystic Lesions

The evaluation of cystic masses is currently the principle application of CEUS in renal pathology. A review of current literature shows the methodology is accepted as the primary imaging technique for the characterization of cystic lesions, with

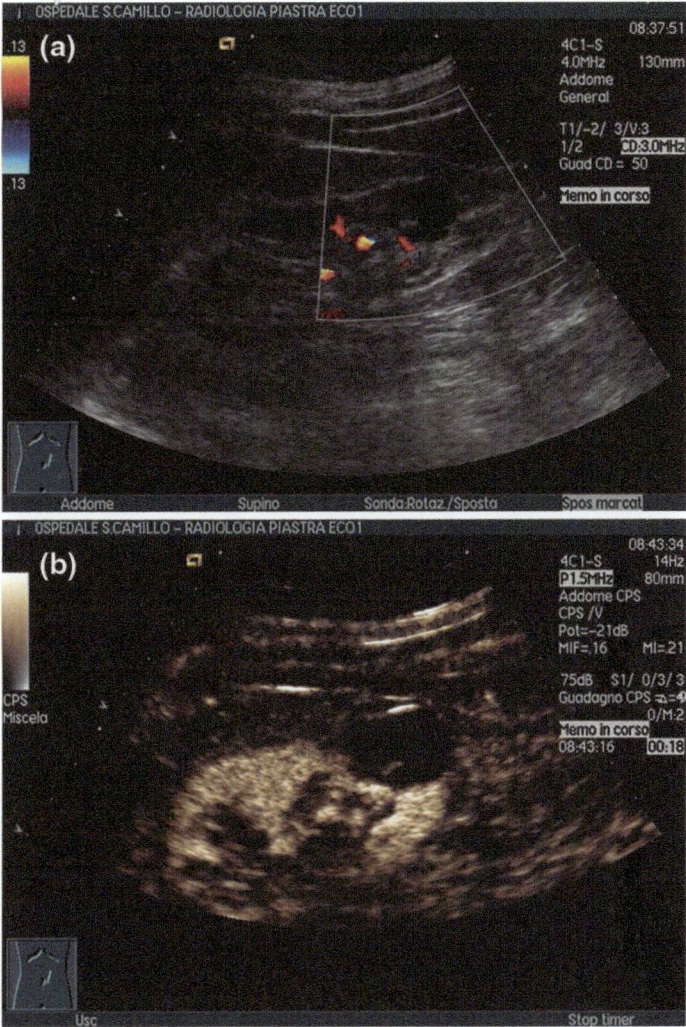

Fig. 2.18 Evaluation of cysts with thin internal septa in baseline examination (**a**) and with CEUS (**b**) which shows no focal thickenings and/or suspicious saturation: cysts of type II according to the Bosniak classification

diagnostic accuracy comparable to that of MSCT [32, 33]; furthermore, the possibility of using CEUS within the Bosniak classification system is now also widely accepted as an alternative to using MSCT [1, 32–34].

A quick review reminds us that Bosniak classification distinguishes five categories, increasing in the degree of possibility of malignancy in the masses identified: Type I and II are characterized by simple cystic formations without calcification and thickening parietal nodules; they may have thin septa without noticeable post-contrast enhancement (Fig. 2.18).

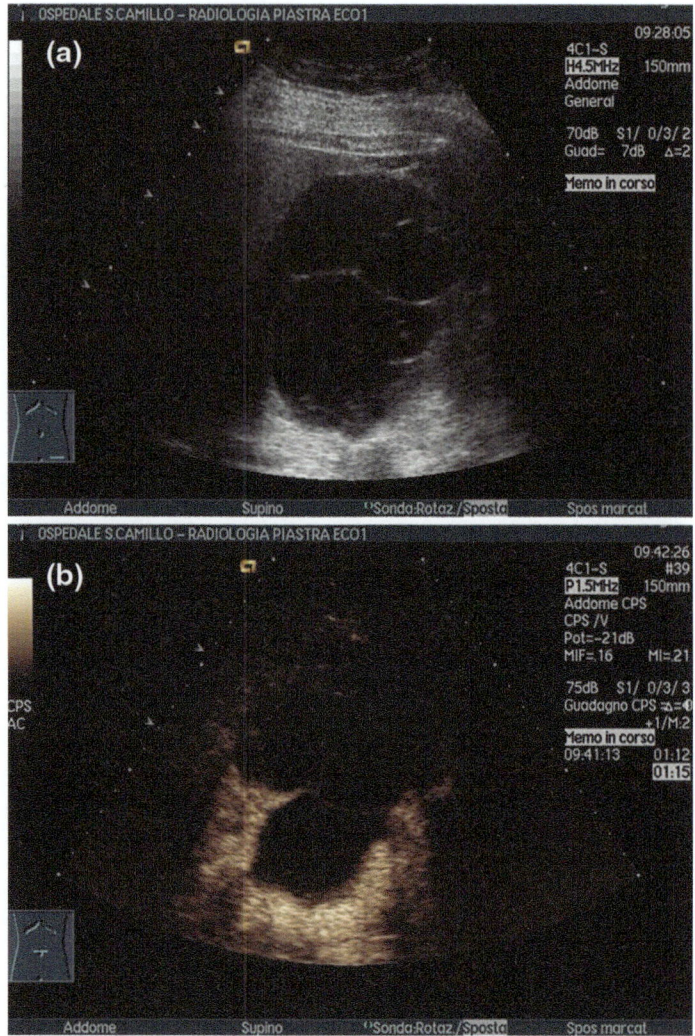

Fig. 2.19 Voluminous cystic formation with multiple internal septa, studied with baseline ultrasound (**a**) and with CEUS (**b**) which shows a discrete enhancement of the septa themselves: a type IIF cyst according to Bosniak classification

Type IIF (where F stands for follow-up) is characterized by the presence of thin septa which are more numerous than in the first types, and possible modest focal thickenings that may show up in a minimal post-contrast enhancement (Fig. 2.19).

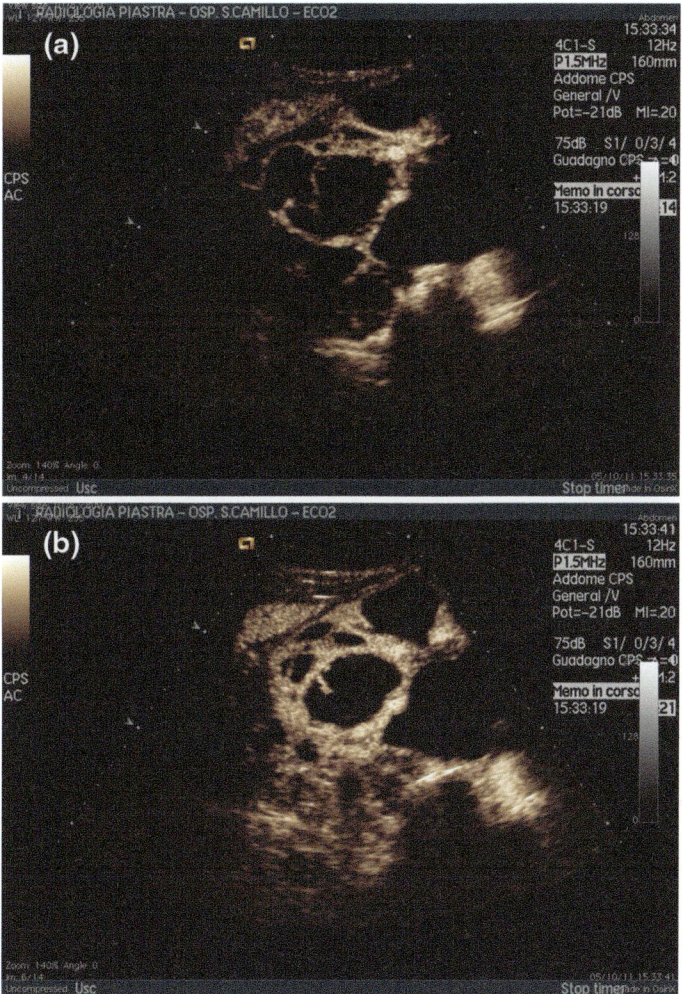

Fig. 2.20 **a–c** Complex cystic lesion with numerous thickened septa and nodules showing in CEUS with high post-contrast enhancement: type III cyst according to Bosniak classification

Types III and IV are distinguished with nodular parietal thickening, calcifications, thick internal septa, with post-contrast enhancement (Fig. 2.20); the two categories differ in that in type IV, the post-contrast enhancement is uneven in all areas of the lesion, and not only in the septa and modules (Fig. 2.21).

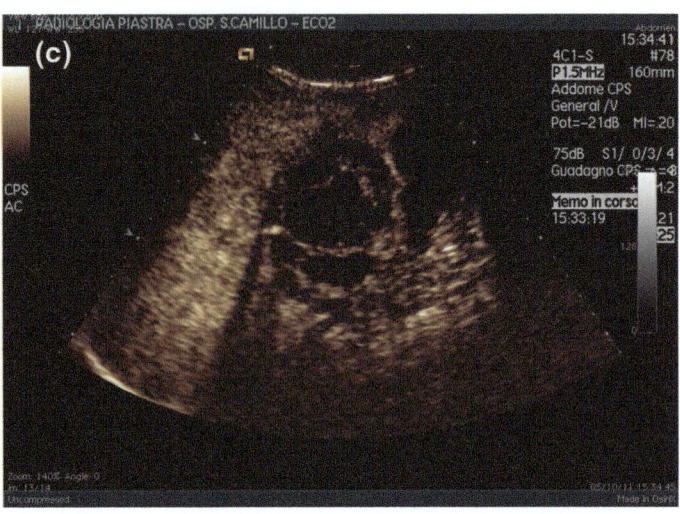

Fig. 2.20 (continued)

The importance of this classification lies in that the types I and II do not require further diagnostic evaluations; type IIF, due to its borderline traits, requires careful follow-up; type III requires a surgical approach for a definitive diagnosis; and membership in type IV makes surgical removal of the formation, which is considered malignant, a necessary step [35].

A ratio has also been discovered which expresses the probability of malignant degeneration in each category: close to 0 % for types I and II, 5 % for type IIF, between 50–70 % for type III, and between 95 and 100 % for type IV [33].

The high diagnostic accuracy, as confirmed by numerous scientific papers, makes it possible to properly treat patients with cystic formations, especially those referred to as complex lesions. In this field, CEUS is to be considered as a second-level test with diagnostic accuracy equal to that of a CT scan and/or MRI, but without the use of nephrotoxic contrast agents or ionizing radiation.

Some authors [36] have reported levels of diagnostic accuracy even higher than that for CT, indicating that the method is effective not only in the characterization of a cystic lesion, but also in the follow-up of progressed lesions such as a type IIF.

Our experience has proven to be in line with that published internationally: in 2010–2011, we evaluated 83 patients with cystic formations which were determined not simple by the baseline ultrasound; subsequent CEUS evaluation based on Bosniak classification identified 53/83 formations classified type I or II, 18/83 type IIF, 7/83 type III and 5/83 type IV. Subsequent evaluation with MSCT scans and/or MRI using of iodinated or paramagnetic contrast media confirmed the capacity of CEUS, as has already been reported in publication [33, 34, 37], to both identify septa nodules smaller than those identified by the other two techniques, and also provide a greater post-contrast enhancement. This second factor allows us to classify lesions that other techniques tend to 'underestimate' in a certain sense

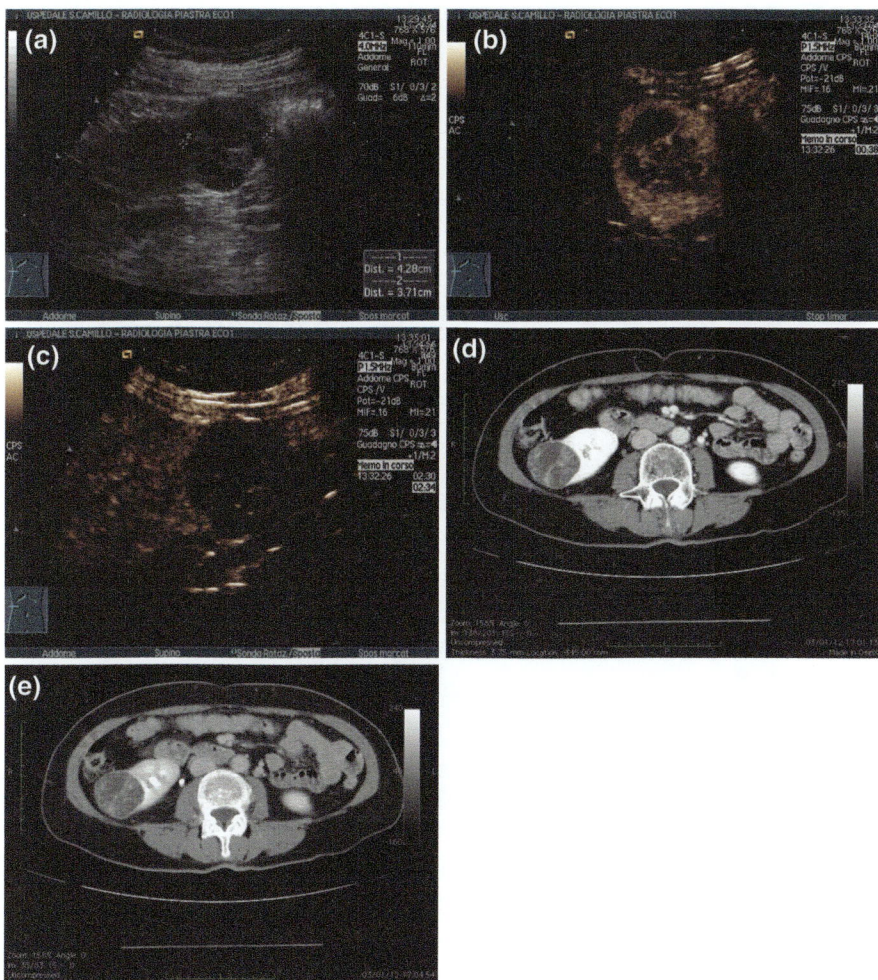

Fig. 2.21 Integrated assessment with baseline ultrasound (**a**), CEUS (**b, c**), and MSCT (**d, e**) of a cystic lesion with saturation both in the septa as well as in other components of the lesion: clear cell adenocarcinoma

in the proper, higher category. This underestimation does not cause great problems in the treatment of patients for types I and II, but has critical consequences one considers there is a real mismatch between the techniques for categories IIF and III. In our experience, this occurred in 3/83 cases which by CEUS were classified as category III, while the MSTC scan had resulted in a classification of category II; following standard clinical/urological assessment (of age, risk factors, good contralateral functionality of the kidney), a histological characterization was carried out which identified 1/3 cases of an evolving lesion.

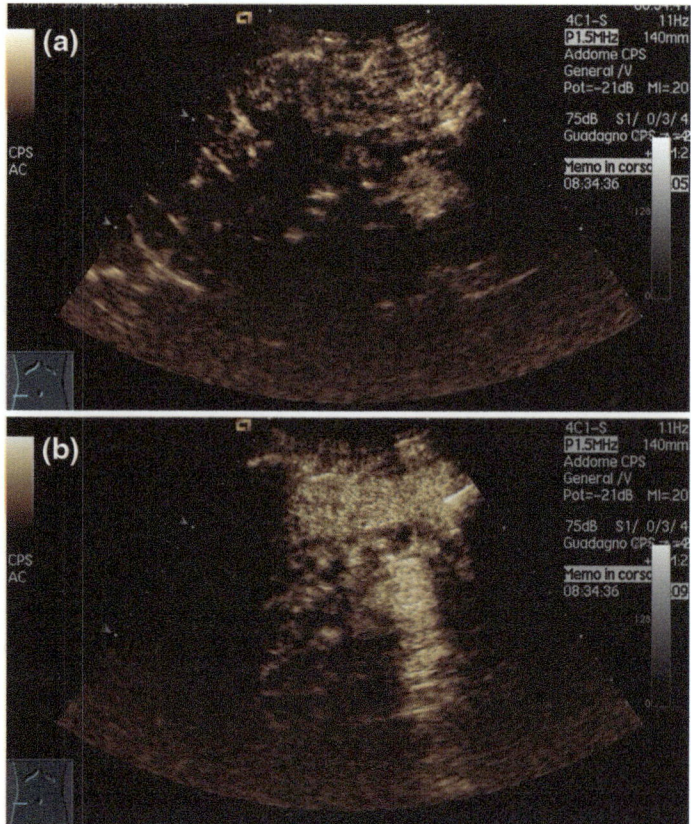

Fig. 2.22 Evaluation of parenchyma in patients with polycystic syndrome, in dialysis for over 5 years. Detection of an expansive formation, with lively post-contrast saturation in the early arterial phase with persistence of the same in the late arterial phase (**a–b**). Evaluation of the same case with multiphase CT scan (**c–d**). Histological evaluation showed the presence of a papillary evolving lesion

CEUS methodology, in our opinion, delivers high diagnostic accuracy, and becomes especially crucial in light of treatment considerations, in order to avoid the repetition of high-strain tests in patients who may already have impaired renal function. For this reason, our procedure for patients whose baseline ultrasound shows a mass with small signs of complexity (evidence that septa are too thin and/or the lack of clear reinforcement of the rear wall), we integrate the examine with the use of second generation CM by IV, and add an MRI targeting the kidney only in the case of persistent doubt. In situations with signs indicating the likelihood of type III or IV classification, we perform a full-body MSCT scan, so as to have both a diagnostic confirmation and accurate staging. CUES appears as the first choice in the monitoring of patients with polycystic syndromes, especially those undergoing dialysis treatments. As is well documented, the association between dialysis and

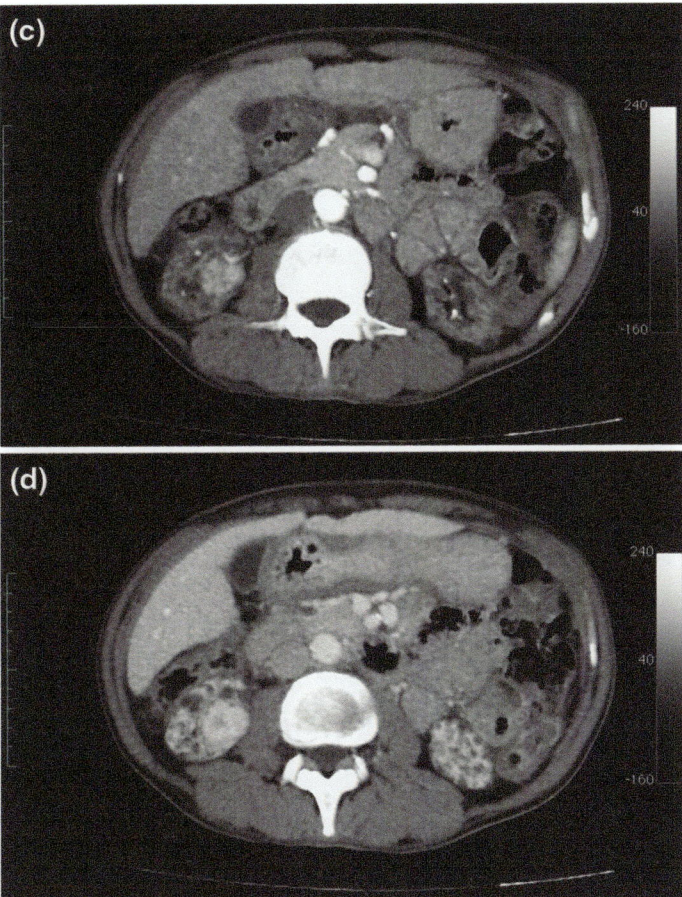

Fig. 2.22 (continued)

polycystic disease can be the cause, in these patients, of a greater likelihood of the development of renal evolving lesions; for this reason, these patients should be monitored for longer periods of time in order to anticipate possible transplant failure. In our work, we have implemented a study protocol that requires an annual CEUS examination in each of the patients referred to our hemodialysis center in order to identify the development of any evolving lesions (Fig. 2.22).

2.7 Pseudomasses

The term pseudomass or pseudotumor indicates a wide variety of anatomical variants which, within the kidney, tend to mimic the traits of an expansive mass [38, 39]. Pseudomasses can be congenital or acquired: included among the first category

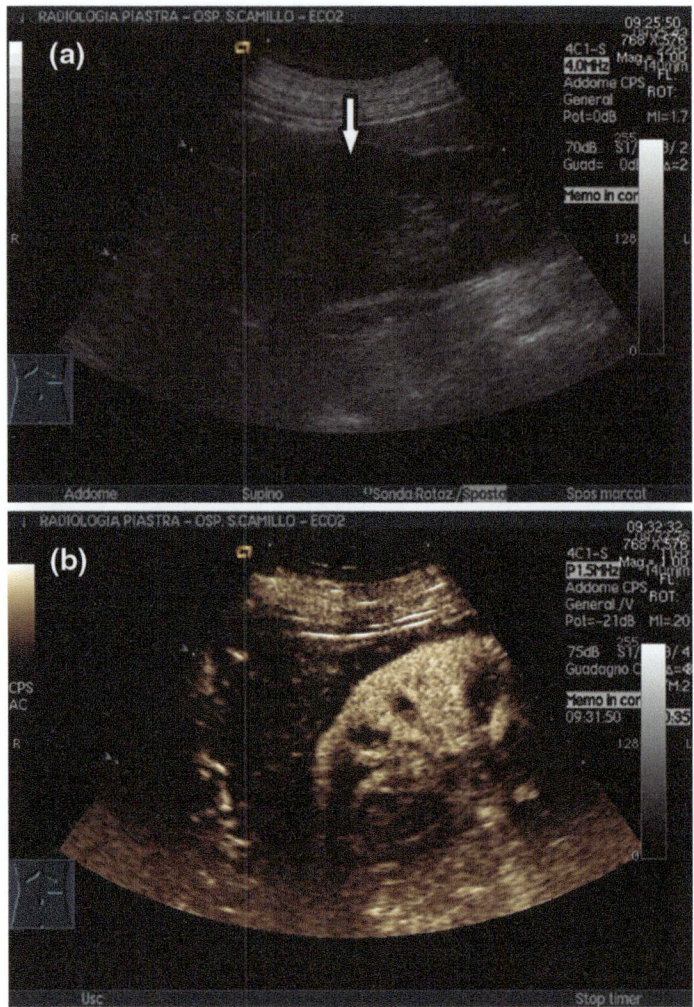

Fig. 2.23 Hypertrophy of the column of Bertin. Evaluation with baseline examination (**a**) and CEUS (**b**), in this case definitive without need for further tests

are hypertrophies of the column of Bertin (Fig. 2.23), prominence of a splenic bump, persistence of fetal lobes (Fig. 2.24) and hilar lip; the second category includes compensatory parenchymal hypertrophy linked to parenchymal retraction. The use of CEUS appears to be nullifying, both in our experience and from what emerged in the literature [24, 40], seeing as the anatomical conditions described above manifest perfusion levels comparable to those of healthy parenchyma, so that

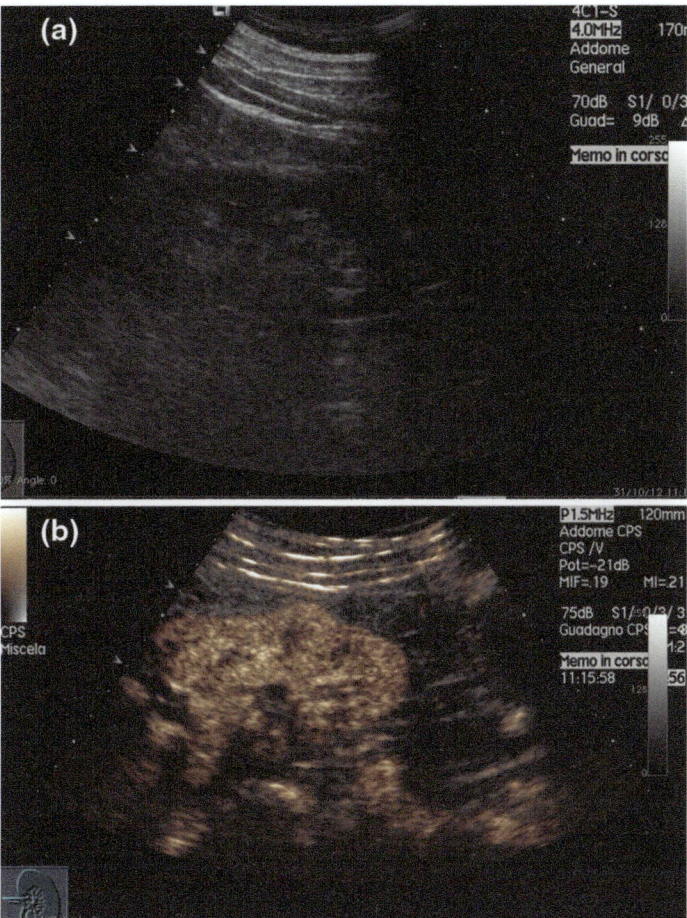

Fig. 2.24 Suspicious baseline examination of nodules in the left kidney (**a**), CEUS evaluation (**b**) does not detect parenchymal changes, showing only a profile lobature. The uro-TC scan with MIP reconstruction (**c**) confirms the finding of the CEUS

in all phases of the CEUS it impossible to discriminate between the pseudo lesion and the surrounding healthy parenchyma. This allows for a reliable diagnosis differentiating pseudo lesions from other expansive forms of kidney lesions of kidney, which, as we have seen in preceding paragraphs, are characterized by CEUS patterns that vary, in comparison with neighboring parenchyma, depending on the phase in which they are evaluated. This application gains a recognized importance when we consider its diagnostic accuracy which seems equivalent to that of other imaging techniques such as CT and/or MRI [24, 40]; consequently, before

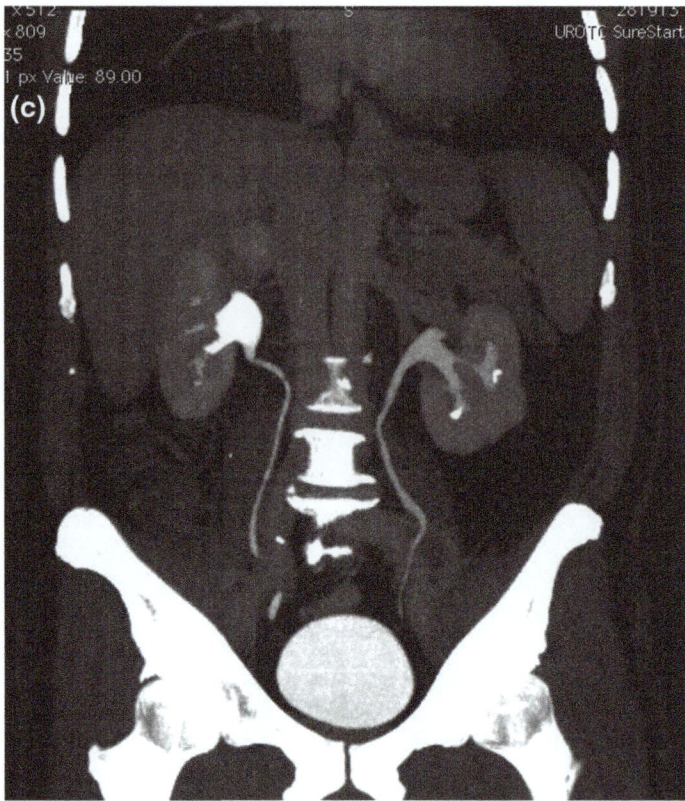

Fig. 2.24 (continued)

subjecting patients to stressful CT or MRI examinations, it is advisable to use a CEUS assessment which may be sufficient, and could prevent unnecessary exposure and economic expense.

References

1. Siracusano S, Bertolotto M, Ciciliato S et al (2011) The current role of contrast-enhanced ultrasound (CEUS) imaging in the evaluation of renal pathology. World J Urol 29:633–638
2. Bertolotto M, Martegani A, Aiani L et al (2008) Value of contrast-enhanced ultrasonography for detecting renal infarcts proven by contrast enhanced CT-a feasibility study. Eur Radiol 18:376–383
3. Nicolau C, Ripollés T (2011) Contrast-enhanced ultrasound in abdominal imaging. Abdom Imaging 37:1–19
4. Setola SV, Catalano O, Sandomenico F, Siani A (2007) Contrastenhanced sonography of the kidney. Abdom Imaging 32:21–28

5. Piscaglia F, Nolsøe C, Dietrich CF et al (2012) The EFSUMB guidelines and recommendations on the clinical practice of Contrast Enhanced Ultrasound (CEUS): update 2011 on non-hepatic applications. Ultraschall Med 33:33–59

6. Valentino M, Serra C, Zironi G et al (2006) Blunt abdominal trauma:emergency contrast-enhanced sonography for detection of solid organ injuries. Am J Roentgenol 186:1361–1367

7. Regine G, Atzori M, Miele V et al (2007) Second-generation sonographic contrast agents in the evaluation of renal trauma. Radiol Med 112:581–587

8. Valentino M, Ansaloni L, Catena F et al (2009) Contrast-enhanced ultrasonography in blunt abdominal trauma: considerations after 5 years of experience. Radiol Med 114:1080–1193

9. Claudon M, Cosgrove D, Albrecht T et al (2008) Guidelines and good clinical practice recommendations for contrast enhanced ultrasound(CEUS), update 2008. Ultraschall Med 29:28–44

10. Sebastia C, Quiroga S, Boyè R et al (2001) Helical CT in renal transplantation: normal findings and early and late complications. Radiographics 21:1103–1117

11. Allan PL, Dubbins PA, Pozniak MA et al (2006) Doppler ultrasoundevaluation of transplantation. In: Allan PL, Dubbins PA, PozniakMA et al (eds) Clinical doppler ultrasound, 2nd edn. Churchill Livingstone Elsevier, Philadelphia

12. Brown ED, Chen MY, Wolfman NT et al (2000) Complications of renal transplantation: evaluation with US and radionuclide imaging. Radiographics 20:607–622

13. Akbar SA, Jafri SZ, Amendola MA et al (2005) Complications of renal transplantation. Radiographics 25:1335–1356

14. Wilson SR, Burns PN (2010) Microbubble-enhanced US in body imaging: what role? Radiology 257:24–39

15. Quaia E (2007) Microbubble ultrasound contrast agents: an update. Eur Radiol 17:1995–2008

16. Schwenger V, Korosoglou G, Hinkel UP et al (2006) Real-time contrast-enhanced sonography of renal transplant recipients predicts chronic allograft nephropathy. Am J Transplant 6:609–615

17. Fontanilla T, Minaya J, Cortes C et al (2012) Acute complicated pyelonephritis: contrast-enhanced ultrasound. Abdom Imaging 37(4):639–646

18. Mitterberger M, Pinggera GM, Colleselli D et al (2008) Acute pyelonephritis: comparison of diagnosis with computed tomography and contrast-enhanced ultrasonography. BJU Int 101:341–344

19. Prakash A, Tan GJ, Wansaicheong GK (2011) Contrast enhanced ultrasound of kidneys. pictorial essay. Med Ultrason 13:150–156

20. Gerst S, Hamm LE, Li D et al (2011) Evaluation of renal masses with contrast-enhanced ultrasound: initial experience. Am J Roentgenol 197:897–906

21. Ignee A, Straub B, Schuessler G et al (2010) Contrast enhanced ultrasound of renal masses. World J Radiol 2:15–31

22. Quaia E, Bussani R, Cova M et al (2005) Radiologic-pathologic correlationsof intratumoral tissue components in the most common solid and cystic renal tumors. pictorial review. Eur Radiol 15:1734–1744

23. Xu HX (2009) Contrast-enhanced ultrasound: the evolving applications. World J Radiol 1:15–24

24. Siracusano S, Quaia E, Bertolotto M et al (2004) The application of ultrasound contrast agents in the characterization of renal tumors. World J Urol 22:316–322

25. Jiang J, Chen Y, Zhou Y, Zhang H (2010) Clear cell renal cell carcinoma:contrast-enhanced ultrasound features relation to tumor size. Eur J Radiol 73:162–167

26. Wink MH, de la Rosette JJ, Laguna P et al (2007) Ultrasonographyof renal masses using contrast pulse sequence imaging: a pilot study. J Endourol 21:466–472

27. Xu ZF, Xu HX, Xie XY et al (2010) Renal cell carcinoma and renal angiomyolipoma: differential diagnosis with real time contrast-enhanced ultrasonography. J Ultrasound Med 29:709–717

28. Fan L, Lianfang D, Jinfang X et al (2008) Diagnostic efficacy of contrast-enhanced ultrasonography in solid renal parenchymal lesions with maximum diameters of 5 cm. J Ultrasound Med 27:875–885
29. Roy C, Gengler L, Sauer B, Lang H (2008) Role of contrast enhanced US in the evaluation of renal tumors. J Radiol 89:1735–1744
30. Tamai H, Takiguchi Y, Oka M et al (2005) Contrast-enhanced ultrasonography in the diagnosis of solid renal tumors. J Ultrasound Med 24:1635–1640
31. Xu ZF, Xu HX, Xie XY et al (2010) Renal cell carcinoma: real timecontrast enhanced ultrasound findings. Abdom Imaging 35:750–756
32. Ascenti G, Mazziotti S, Zimbaro G et al (2007) Complex cystic renal masses:characterization with contrast-enhanced. Radiology 243:158–165
33. Nicolau C, Bunesch L, Sebastia C (2011) Renal complex cysts in adults: contrast-enhanced ultrasound. Abdom Imaging 36:742–752
34. Park BK, Kim B, Kim SH et al (2007) Assessment of cystic renal masses based on Bosniak classification: comparison of CT and contrast-enhanced US. Eur J Radiol 61:310–314
35. Israel GM, Bosniak MA (2005) How i do it: evaluating renal masses. Radiology 236:441–450
36. Quaia E, Bertolotto M, Cioffi V et al (2008) Comparison of contrast-enhanced sonography with unenhanced sonography and contrast-enhanced CT in the diagnosis of malignancy in complex cystic renal masses. Am J Roentgenol 191:1239–1249
37. Clevert DA, Minaifar N, Weckbach S et al (2008) Multislice computed tomography versus contrast-enhanced ultrasound in evaluation of complex cystic renal masses using the Bosniak classification system. Clin Hemorheol Microcirc 39:171–178
38. Bhatt S, MacLennan G, Dogra V (2007) Renal pseudotumors. Am J Roentgenol 188: 1380–1387
39. Regine G, Atzori M, Danza FM (2010) Malformazioni del rene edelle vie urinary. In: Blandino A, Danza FM, Menchi I et al (eds) Imaging dell'apparato urogenitale. Springer, Milano, pp 13–24
40. Mazziotti S, Zimbaro F, Pandolfo A et al (2010) Usefulness of contrast-enhanced ultrasonography in the diagnosis of renal pseudotumors. Abdom Imaging 35:241–245

Urinary Tract and Bladder

3

As has already been stated in describing the chemical and physical properties of the sulfur hexafluoride microbubble [1, 2], it has no excretion through the emunctory kidney. Though this means the advantage that it can be used in patients with reduced renal functionality, from the diagnostic point of view it presents a limit in the detection of urothelial lesions in the calicopyelic and ureteral regions. In fact, the presence of new urothelial formations within the kidney may be suspect when accompanied by hydronephrosis or when a mass is detected with infiltrative growth into the parenchyma: compared to the baseline sonogram, CEUS can more accurately identify the presence of a lesion with heterogeneous and variable post-contrast enhancement (Fig. 3.1), when combined with calyceal dilatation or of the renal pelvis (Fig. 3.2); but it does not provide a reliable determination if it belongs to the urinary excretory system. For this reason, the uroCT (urographic CT) or the uroMRI (urographic MRI) turn out to be the methods of choice (Fig. 3.3).

For bladder injuries, a number of published studies [3, 4] used the CEUS method for both the detection and for the definition of the T parameter in staging. It is in fact fundamental to define the degree of encroachment of the lesion, as the infiltration of the muscular tunic means directing the patient towards cystectomy, while more superficial forms can be treated with endoscopic resection, with or without the localized administration of chemotherapeutic agents [3].

These studies have shown that it is possible, through the use of contrast media, to differentiate the various layers of the bladder wall [3]: in fact, both the mucosa and the submucosa show rapid post-contract saturation which persists for about 1–2 min, unlike the muscular layer which shows lesser and more delayed saturation; tumors have a lively post-contrast enhancement at an early stage, which persists in the later stages (Fig. 3.4). This behavior allows for better diagnostic accuracy in detection with CEUS compared to a baseline sonogram, and can be used to determine whether or not there is encroachment into the muscle layer (Fig. 3.5) [3, 4]. The limits of the technique are found in the evaluation of lesions that appear flat, from columnar hypertrophia of the bladder wall linked to a

G. Regine et al., *Contrast-Enhanced Ultrasound of the Urinary Tract*,
DOI: 10.1007/978-88-470-5432-5_3, © Springer-Verlag Italia 2013

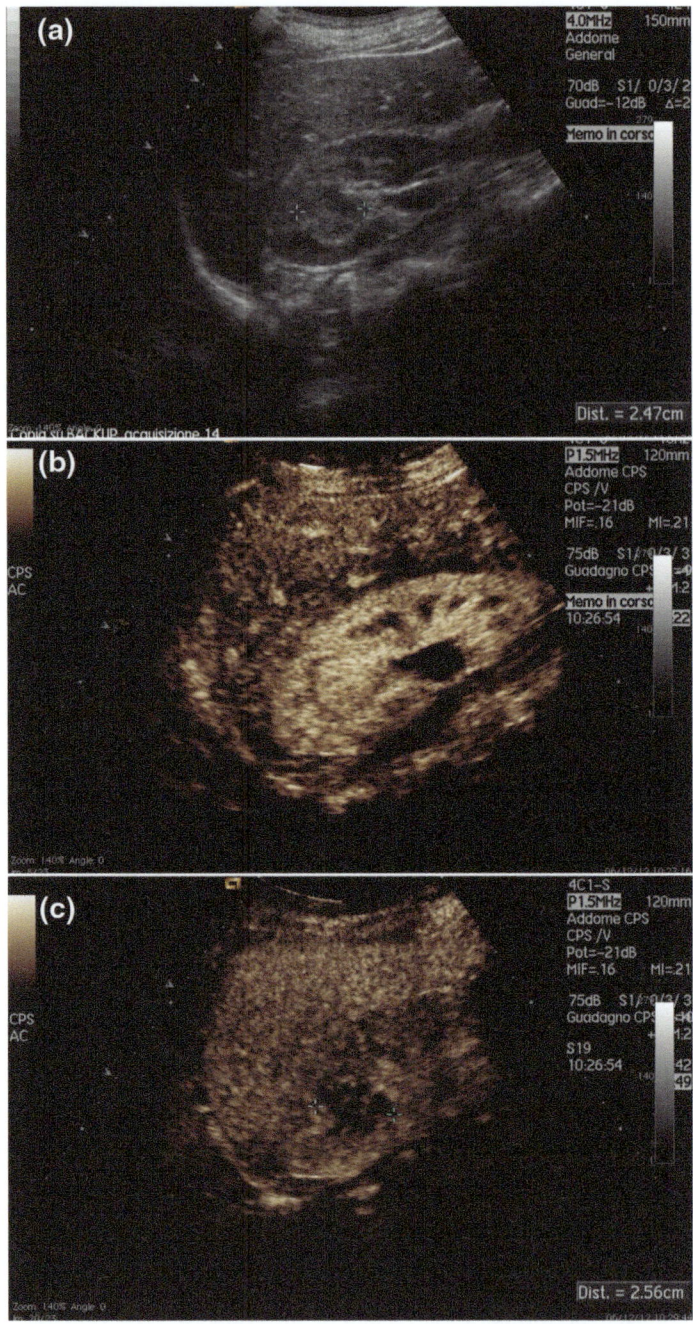

Fig. 3.1 Integrated assessment with baseline ultrasound, CEUS, and uro CT showing expansive lesion infiltrating the upper calyceal group of the right kidney. In CEUS, the solid nodule identified in the baseline examination (**a**) shows high wash-in in the early phase (**b**) with subsequent wash-out in parenchymal phase (**c**) confirmation of that finding on a late uroTC scan (**d**); the urographic MIP 3D reconstruction documents an amputated appearance in the same calyceal group (**e**). Urothelial lesions of the upper calyx of the right kidney

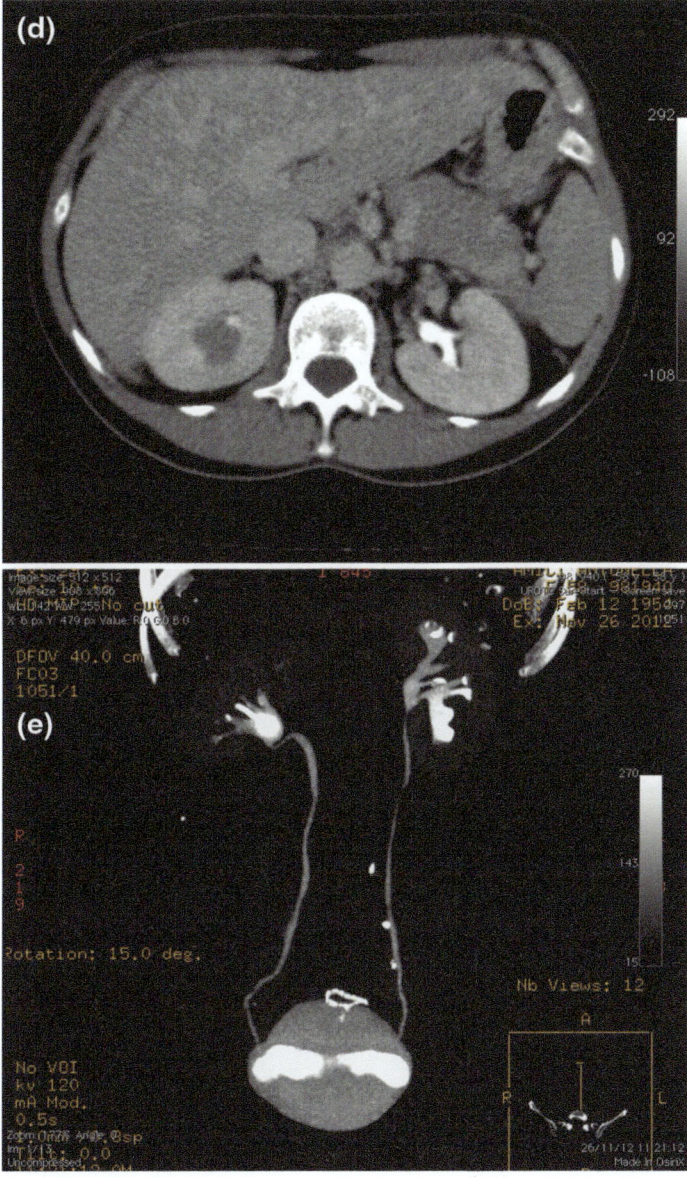

Fig. 3.1 (continued)

condition of prostatic hypertrophy; as well as the limitations inherent to that technique (it is always necessary to perform the examination with adequate intravesical refilling). Our experience targeting this type of application consisted of 39 patients with suspected single and/or multiple bladder lesions who

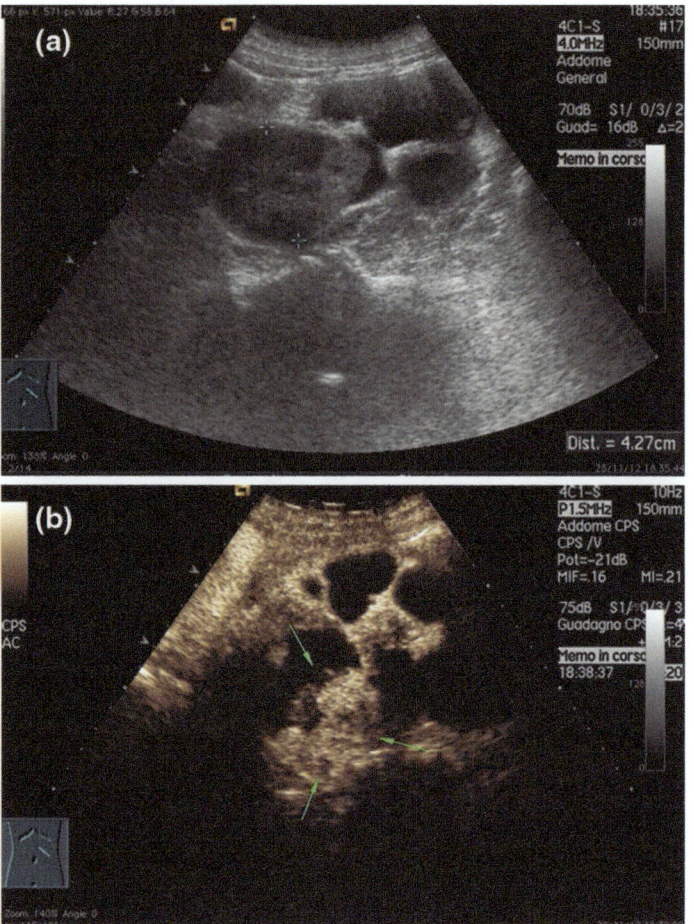

Fig. 3.2 Voluminous lesion of the left renal pelvis assessed by baseline (**a**) and CEUS (**b**) with identification of an expansive formation showing uneven saturation (*arrows*), indicating a marked hydronephrosis

underwent baseline ultrasound tests, CEUS, MRI and/or uroCT, and subsequent cystoscopic evaluation in cases that were positive cases or in which there were doubts. Out of a total of 51 lesions defined by cystoscopy, CEUS identified 46/51 lesions, all larger than 5 mm, while MRI identified 51/51; in the 46 lesions identified, CEUS (ultrasound using contrast media) showed in 23/46 cases an affected muscular tunic; MRI, of the 51 diagnosed, found 27 cases affecting the muscular tunic, while staging cystoscopy identified 25. Two cases of suspected lesions identified by CEUS resulted from sectoral parietal thickenings in a condition of bladder stress properly defined by MRI integrated with use of diffusion-weighted sequences with values of $b = 800$ and $b = 1000$, with cystoscopic

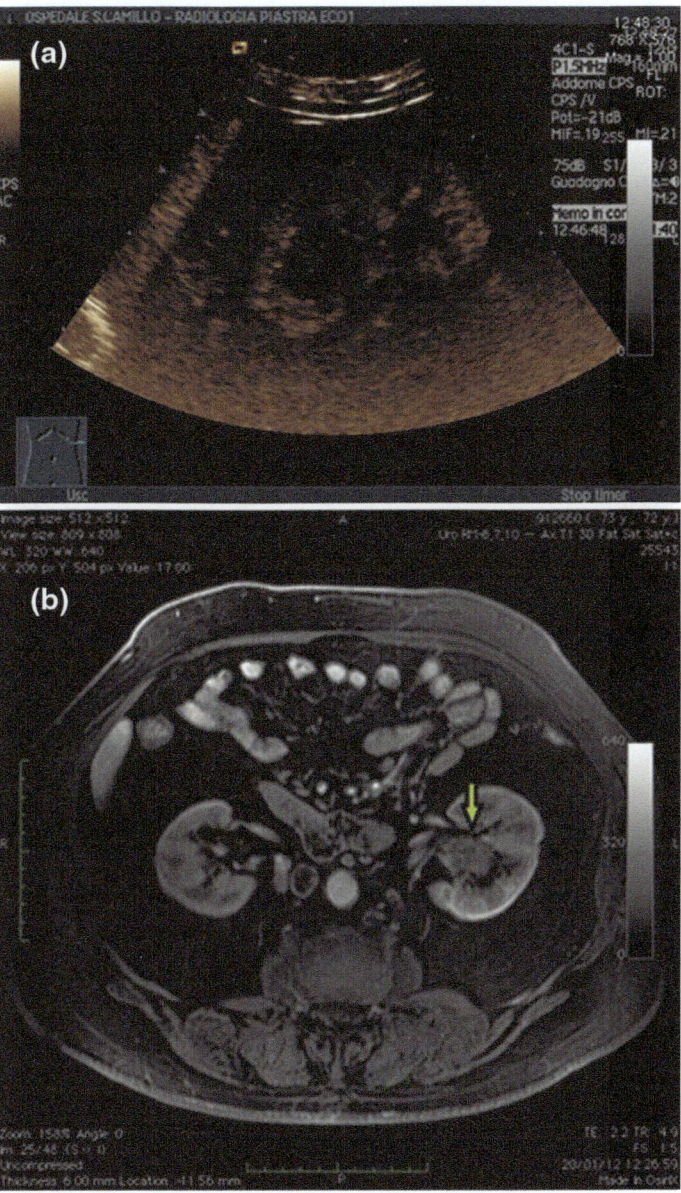

Fig. 3.3 Urothelial lesion of the upper calyceal group and the pelvis of the left kidney, evaluated with CEUS (**a**), which shows calyceal dilation, with a cloudy region of internal tissue; and with MRI (**b**) after IV infusion of paramagnetic contrast agent, which clearly displays the mass and the hydrocalyx (*arrows*)

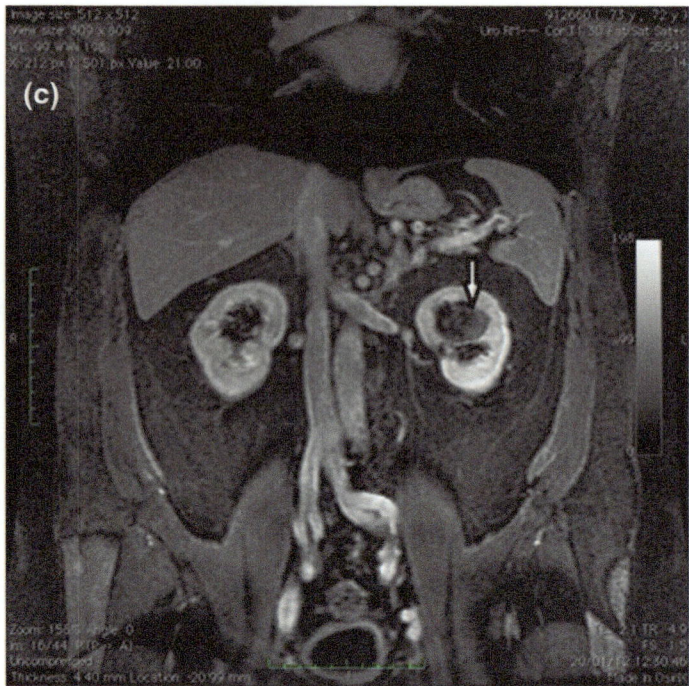

Fig. 3.3 (continued)

confirmation that were therefore not counted in the previous series. In one case, both CEUS and MRI correctly identified and defined the origin of an extravesical lesion on the urachus, which had infiltrated the wall of the bladder dome (Fig. 3.6).

In our opinion, this method appears to be extremely reliable in cases of projecting polypoidal lesions with a broad-based attachment and dimensions larger than 5 mm. It is currently less reliable than MRI for the definition of the T parameter, especially if the lesion is located at the level of the bladder base.

Conversely, we noticed a remarkable accuracy in the definition of the same parameter with respect to baseline ultrasound.

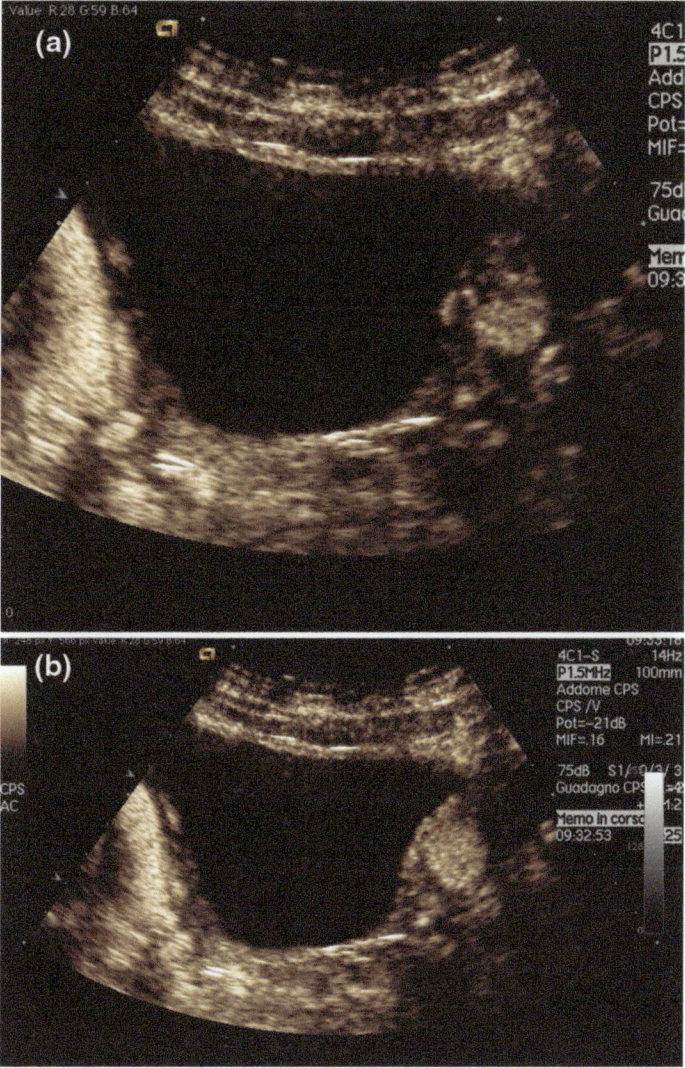

Fig. 3.4 Neoplastic lesion within a diverticular formation of the left bladder wall. Sonogram in early and late phase (**a–b**) and multiphase CT scan (**c–d**) with a detectable highly vascularized lesion affecting the entire diverticular cavity and infringement beyond the muscular tunic

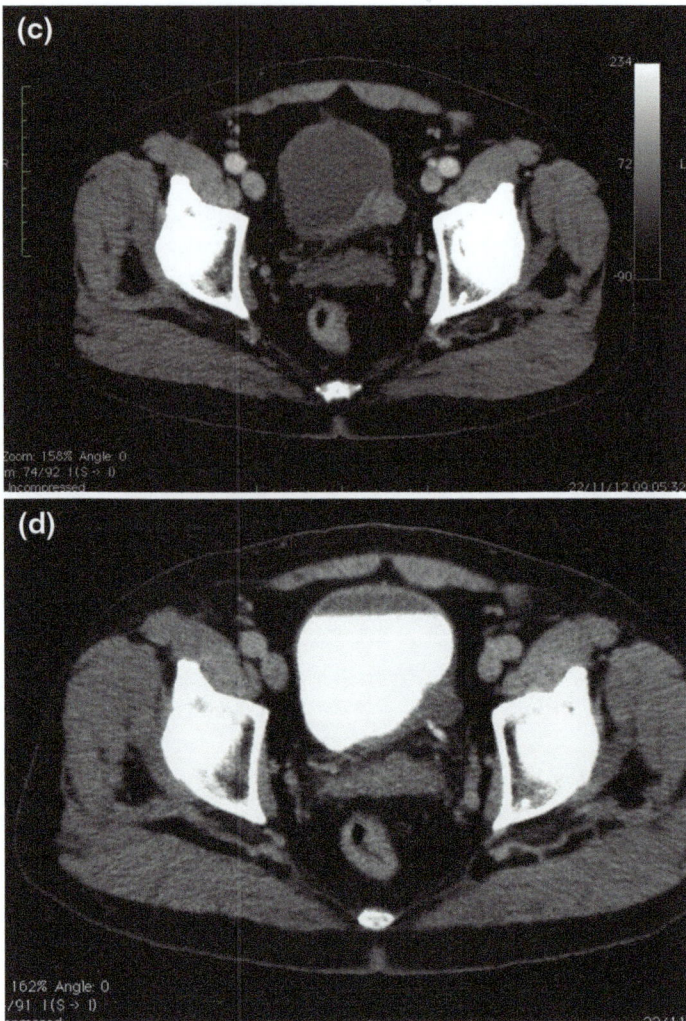

Fig. 3.4 (continued)

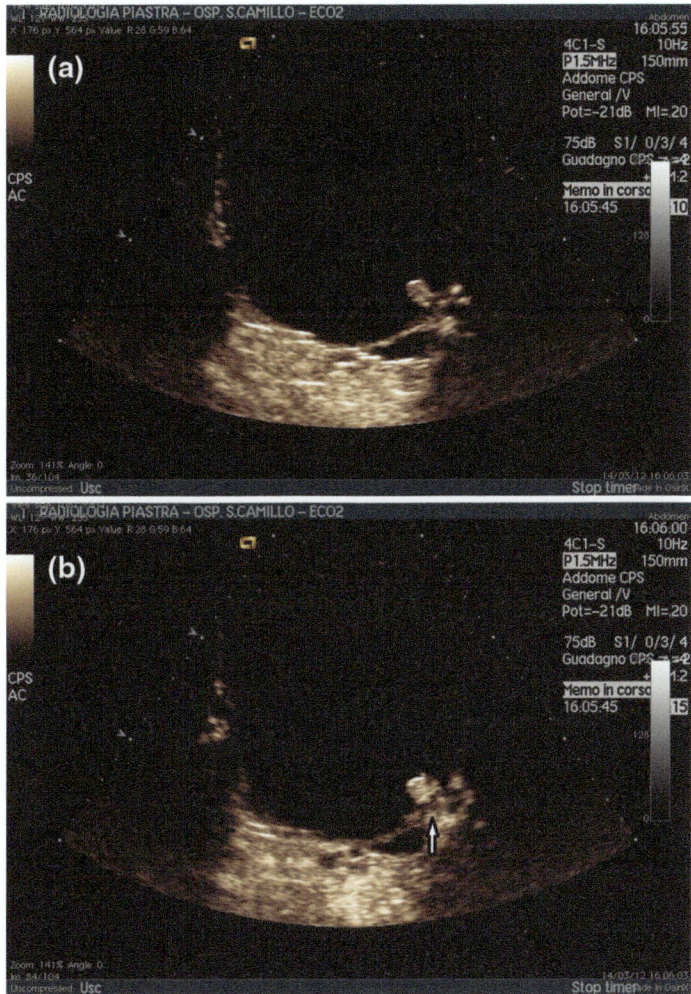

Fig. 3.5 Projecting lesion that shows high saturation during the arterial (**a**) and late (**b**) phases, with a good view of the integrity of the muscular layer of the bladder wall (*arrow*)

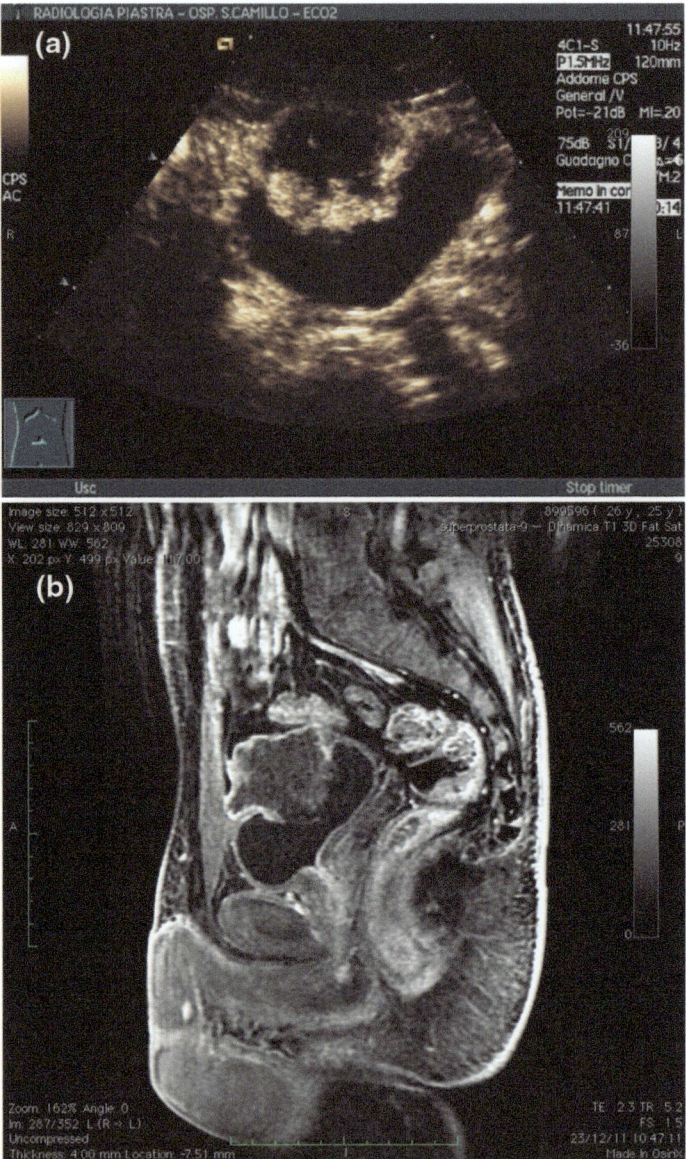

Fig. 3.6 Integrated assessment with CEUS (**a**) and MRI (**b**, **c**) of an extravesical lesion infiltrating the bladder wall: urachal adenocarcinoma

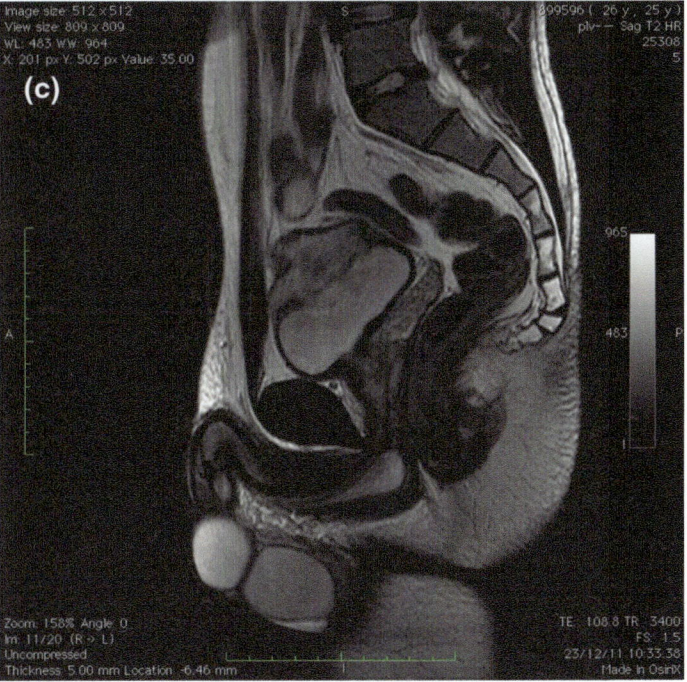

Fig. 3.6 (continued)

References

1. Quaia E (2007) Microbubble ultrasound contrast agents: an update. Eur Radiol 17:1995–2008
2. Piscaglia F, Nolsøe C, Dietrich CF et al (2012) The EFSUMB guidelines and recommendations on the clinical practice of contrast enhanced ultrasound (CEUS): update 2011 on nonhepatic applications. Ultraschall Med 33:33–59
3. Nicolau C, Bunesch L, Peri L et al (2010) Accuracy of contrast enhanced ultrasound in the detection of bladder cancer. Br J Radiol 84:1091–1099
4. Caruso G, Salvaggio G, Campisi A et al (2010) Bladder tumor staging: comparison of contrast-enhanced and gray-scale ultrasound. AJR Am J Roentgenol 194:151–156

MC in Pediatric Ultrasound and in the Study of Vesicoureteral Reflux: "Cystosonography"

4

Ultrasound contrast agent introduced into the bladder is a viable alternative to radiological contrast in the evaluation of ureteral reflux and in the evaluation of the child. It can easily be used to identify the contrast that may flow back into the kidneys.

We have been using cystosonography for several years (Fig. 4.1) in the evaluation of urinary tract infections to detect and quantify vesicoureteral reflux. This as an alternative to the traditional voiding cystourethrogram X-ray (VCUG) (Fig. 4.2) [6] for both the first diagnosis and in regular check-ups after operations. An essential requirement is the availability of an ultrasound with a contrast module, such as the CPS Siemens (Siemens Medical Solutions USA Inc., Mountain View, CA). Due to the uniqueness of the application, we report our specific experience with highlighted technical and semiotic details.

4.1 Cystosonography: Instructions for Use

The contrast agent is the same that has been used for years in systemic intravenous administration. It is called SonoVue (sulfur hexafluoride) (Bracco International B.V. Amsterdam, Netherlands), a drug that has been used for a many years in the study of focal lesions in adults, but is not registered for pediatric use or for intravesical intracavitary administration. This poses the problems of off label use [2, 5, 10] with the necessary authorization the Ethics Committee, of the use of a detailed informed consent and a clear explanation and discussion with the parents. In our experience, there was only one case in which a mother refused the ultrasound examination; while almost every parent was quite happy in proceeding and in avoiding X-rays. In fact, many parents turn to us in order to avoid the use of radiographic exams (VCUG).

G. Regine et al., *Contrast-Enhanced Ultrasound of the Urinary Tract*,
DOI: 10.1007/978-88-470-5432-5_4, © Springer-Verlag Italia 2013

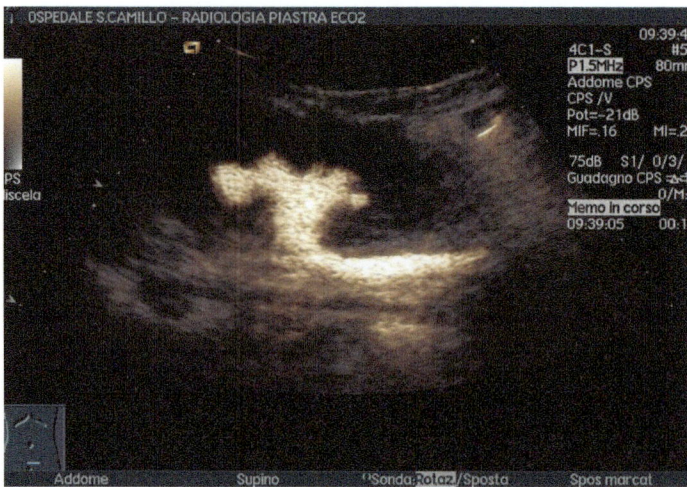

Fig. 4.1 Cistosonography in the study of reflux. Vesicoureteral reflux on the left of second degree: the contrast was evident from along the ureter to the renal cavity

Fig. 4.2 Evaluation of reflux by cystourethrography. Reflux grade 1 on the right and third degree on left

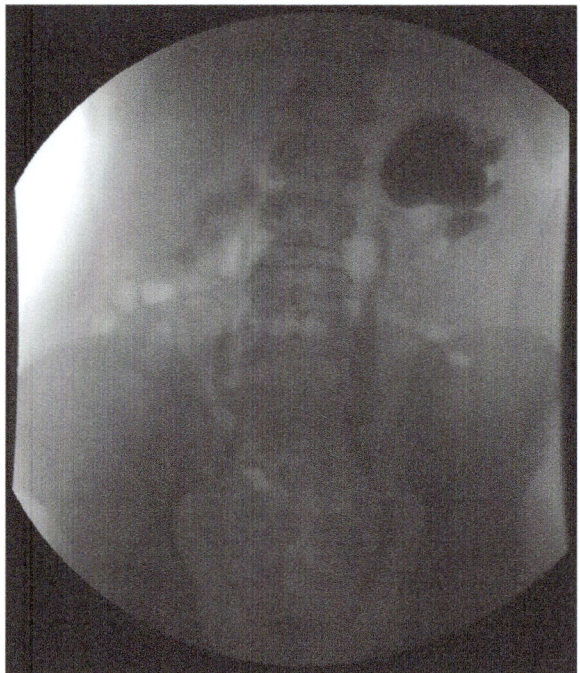

These are all cases of children in which clinical evaluation and sonogram study have been completed, in which the question of reflux is decisive, and conversely a urethral disorder has been ruled out.

The preparation of a child for cystosonography is identical to that for radio-logical cystography. Both cases begin with the placement of a vesical catheter to inject the contrast dye. It proceeds with partial vesical filling using saline solution; evaluating the bladder and distal ureters during that filling (the catherized bladder is almost always empty). Immediately after the introduction 1–1.5 cc of SonoVue, the vesical filling with saline solution resumes, up to the point of urination around the catheter; following this the catheter is removed and a second urination is awaited. During this process, in addition to assessing the refluxes and their size, one can attempt to assess the urethra. The study of the male urethra can be difficult, though dilations and by valve stenosis can be easily detected.

Over a period of 28 months (September 2009–December 2011), we performed 145 cystosonograms and 57 voiding cystourethrograms (VCUG) in infants and children between 3 months and 15 years (mean age 2.5 years). Twenty-eight children underwent both the cystosonogram and VCUG, although at different times.

The cystosonogram has always clearly shown vesicoureteral reflux in grades 2–5. Often, grade 1 refluxes were also evident (in any case clinically insignificant), since even a small number of microbubbles can clearly be seen in the ureter and in the proximal renal pelvis (Fig. 4.3) [1]. In our experience over several years, cystosonogram has allowed us to obtain an accurate diagnosis even in unclear or clinically complex cases. For example, in cases with small reflux or those hard to detect in a refluxing megaureter (Fig. 4.4), in the case of reflux in small kidneys (Fig. 4.5), as well as in the case of double district, with good evidence of refluxing both in the lower district first and then in the other (Fig. 4.6). Another special case

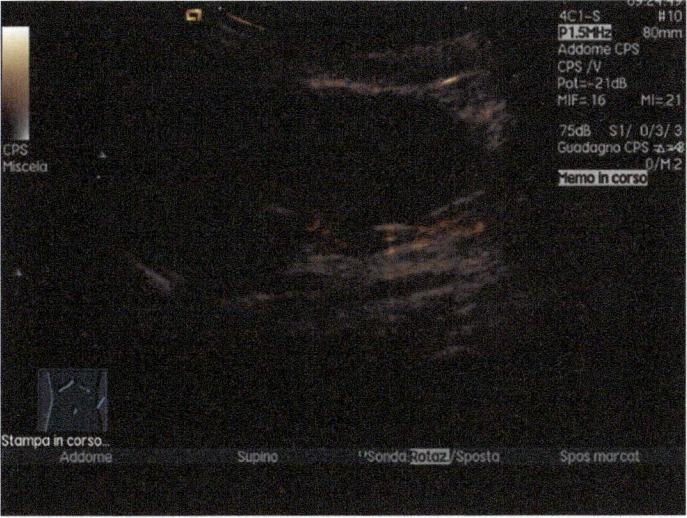

Fig. 4.3 Grade 1 reflux. The CPS module also shows a small amount of contrast material originating from the ureter and reaching the kidney

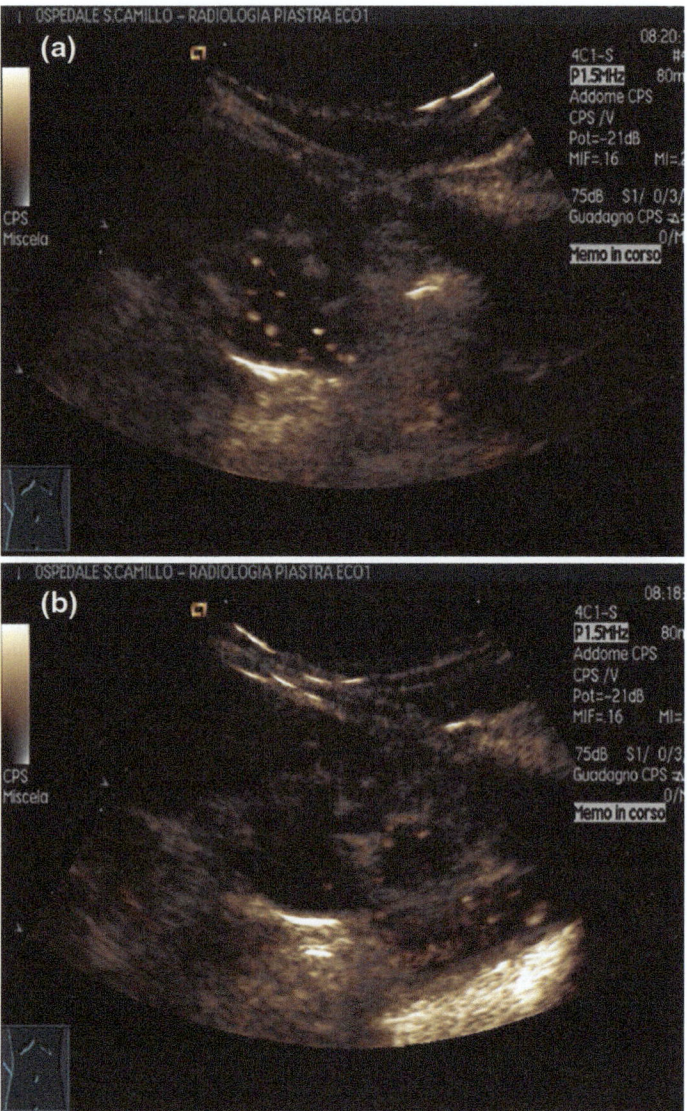

Fig. 4.4 Refluxing megaureter: mild reflux, in wide ureter, and pelvis. Clearly evident are various microbubbles of contrast in the pelvis (**a**) and in the proximal ureter (**b**)

observed was noticed in a check-up after bilateral lateral STING (Subureteral Tetrafluoroethylene Injection) in a child with high-grade reflux: on the right reflux is still present, while on the left the STING determined pyelic expansion without reflux (Fig. 4.7).

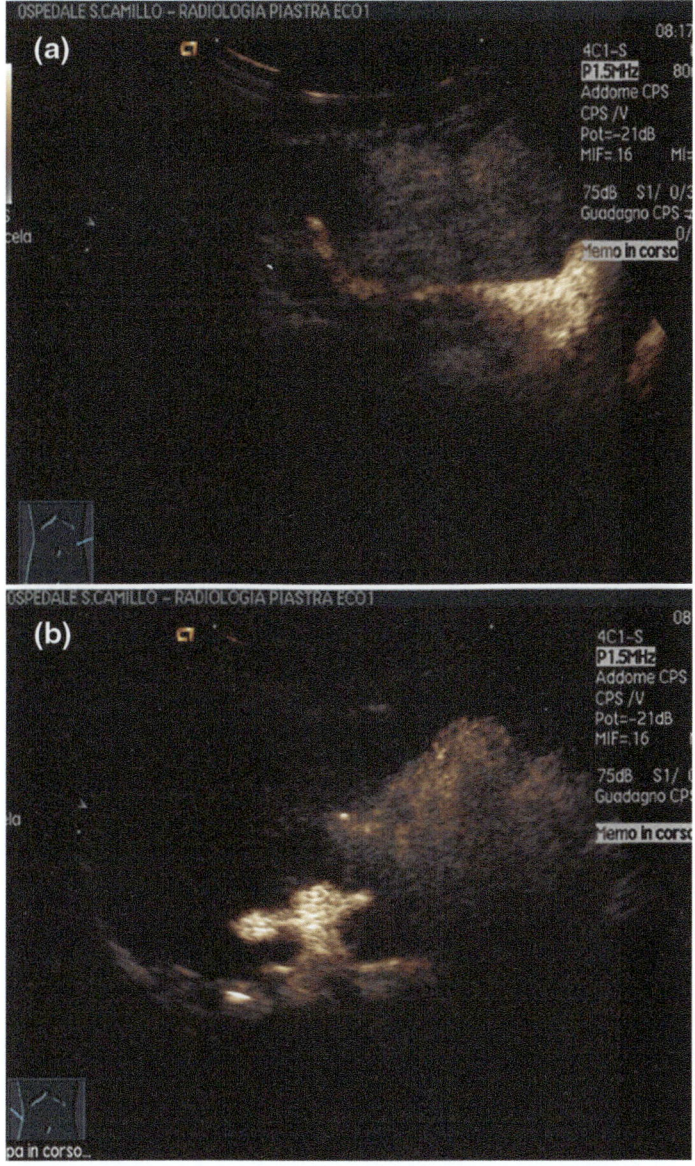

Fig. 4.5 Reflux in the small left kidney, likely outcomes of pyelonephritis (**a**). Reflux also present on the right kidney (**b**)

In the children undergoing follow-up, in 6 cases the first check-up was completed using cystosonography and the second using VCUG. In the other 23 cases (generally boys), the first check-up was radiographic (VCUG) and the second with

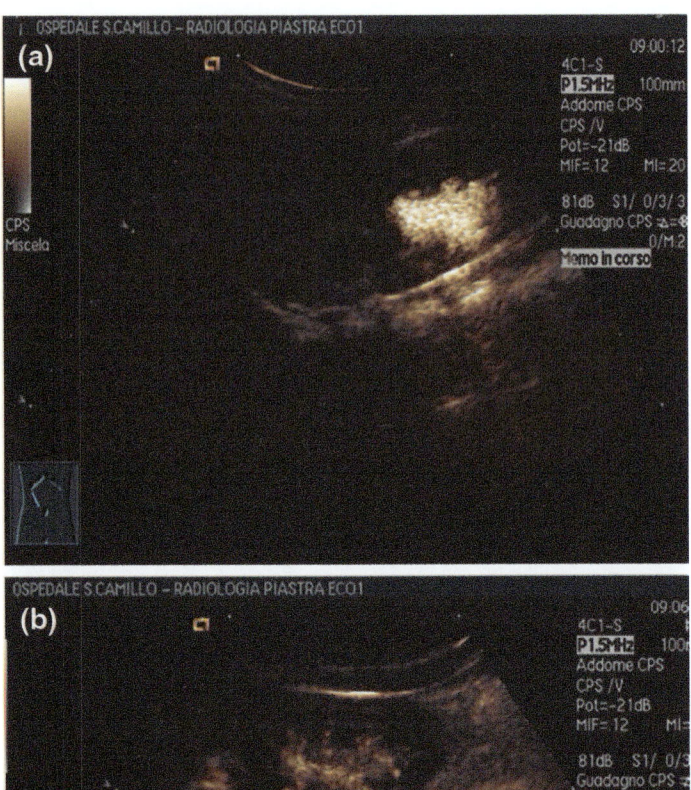

Fig. 4.6 Cistosonography (**a**, **b**) which shows reflux in right double district: reflux first in the lower group, and subsequently also in the upper. Cystography (**c**, **d**) of the same case, with two right double districts and bilateral reflux

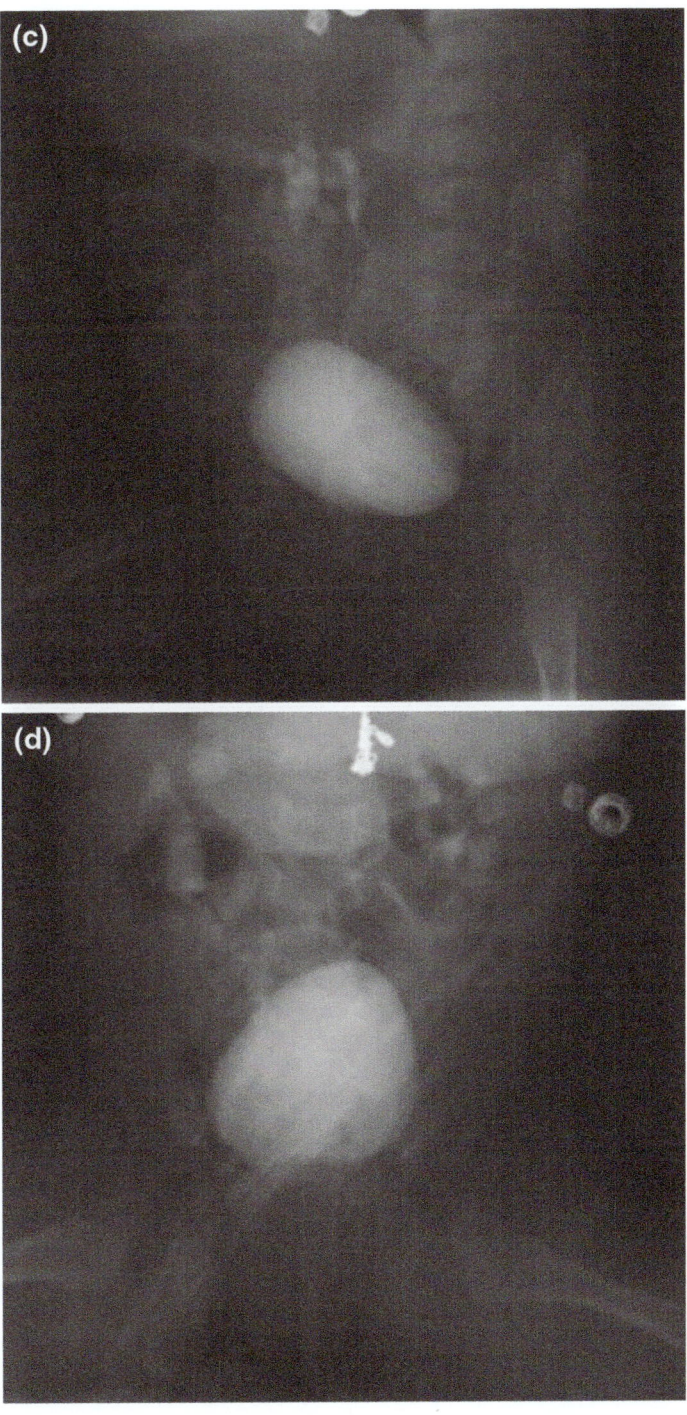

Fig. 4.6 (continued)

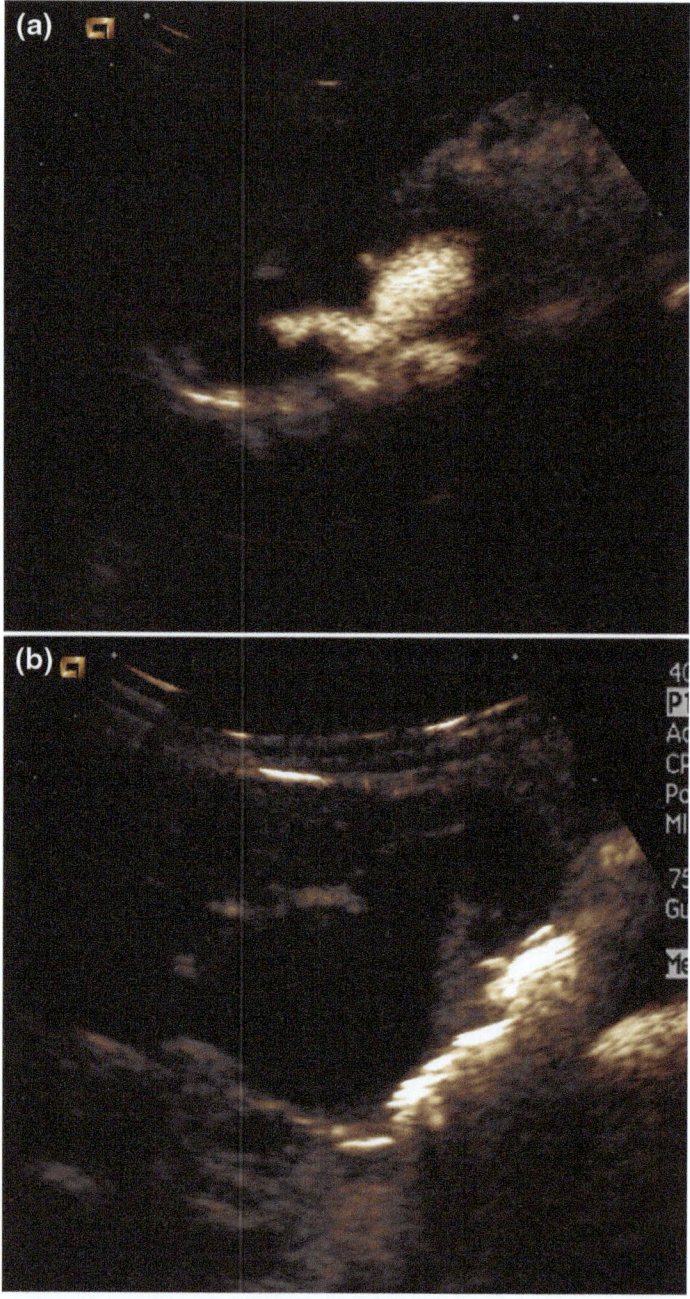

Fig. 4.7 Check-up after bilateral STING: persistence in the right kidney of third degree reflux (**a**). Left kidney reflux disappears, but there remains a residual dilatation (**b**)

cystosonography. Between the two groups there does not appear to be any significant differences in sensitivity to the pathology.

The method is particularly suitable for children when recurrence is suspected after STING interventions in cystoscopy, which is currently the first choice of procedure. These children have recurrent reflux after the first few months of wellbeing; which is because in the initial phase the edema of the submucosal injection keeps the ureterovesicular junction contained, while after 4–10 months it is reduced bringing the possible occurrence of relapses which necessitate another operation.

In our study protocol, cystosonogram is also indicated as the first diagnosis in girls or in boys with unilateral dilatation of the urinary tract. The use of VCUG is preferred when a panoramic view of the bladder is needed, as in the cases of neurogenic bladder; or in a male newborn infant with dilation of both renal pelvises, with the suspected presence of urethral disease urethral which is more visible radiologically. The radiological VCUG exam is much more detailed in the diagnosis of the valves of the urethra or of the syringocele.

We have never observed adverse reactions to the drug during or after cystosonography. The cystosonogram proves to have similar sensitivity to VCUG in the diagnosis of reflux in children [3]; it allows for exploration of the kidneys longer than in X-ray fluoroscopy and has a lower cost since the ionic iodated contrast first used for VCUG is now not available in the market [9]. In addition, it is better accepted by parents and avoids radiation exposure, which is particularly dangerous in children [4]. An obstacle to the spread of the method is the absence of registration for pediatric use of the drug. The informed consent required from the parents is therefore more complicated and a preliminary interview is therefore needed. Also essential is the approval of the Ethics Committee of the hospital.

4.2   Study of Focal Hepatic or Renal Lesions

The use of contrast-enhanced ultrasound in pediatric pathology allows us to avoid the more invasive pediatric exams requiring the use of radiation or sedation [7]. Furthermore, the drug has neither the limitations nor the risks of gadolinium or iodinated contrast in children with renal failure [10, 11, 12].

For example, it may be recommended for the evaluation of liver nodules, to clarify doubts in renal lesions [7] or to detect traumatic lesions on the liver and spleen [2, 10].

The problem of the absence of registration of use of the drug in children remains, but, after an interview, almost all parents give their consent. Otherwise, the alternative is radiation, whether with iodinated contrast agent or gadolinium, and often the sedation of the infant [8]. With a proper clinical diagnosis, laboratory comparison, and possible later distance check-ups, CEUS is often sufficient to answer the query faced by the radiologist.

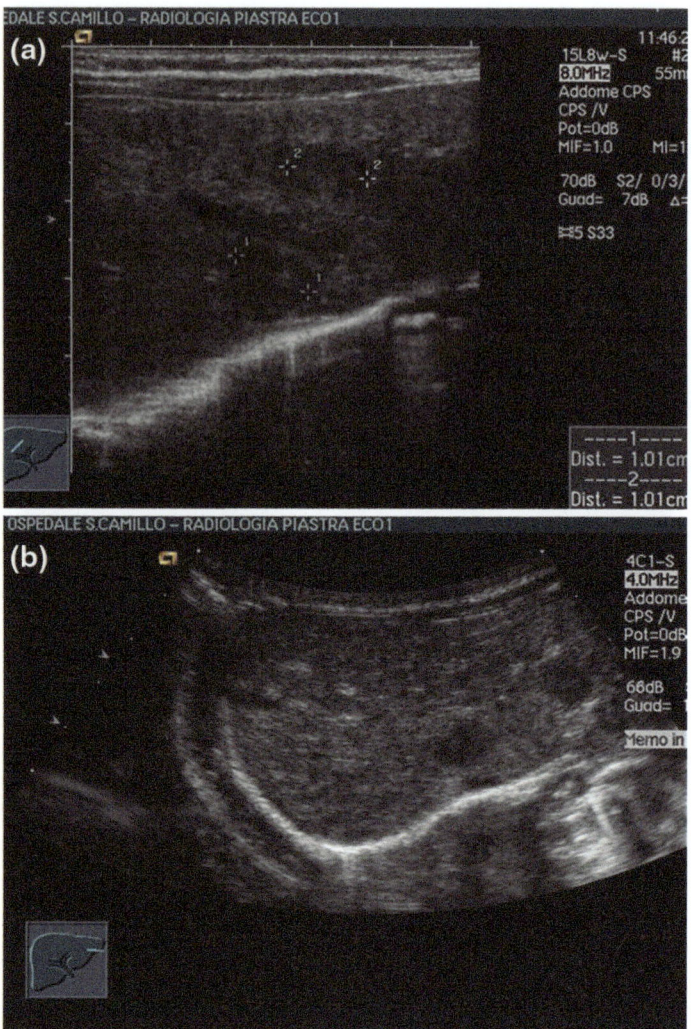

Fig. 4.8 a–b Baseline ultrasound in the course of screening for polycystic kidney disease, which reveals the presence of several nodules within a hepatic region that is mildly echogenic

We have collected a few cases, with the caution imposed by the use of intravenous drugs not registered for pediatrics. These are in any case indicative of the possibilities of the methodology and for its future development in pediatrics.

The first case is an infant a few days old, which had some focal lesions on the hepatic parenchyma; they were noticed by chance in the course of renal ultrasound screening for hip dysplasia (Fig. 4.8a, b). The neonatologist asked us to do a contrast MRI with sedation and to propose a diagnosis, particularly deciding whether or not we could exclude hepatoblastoma.

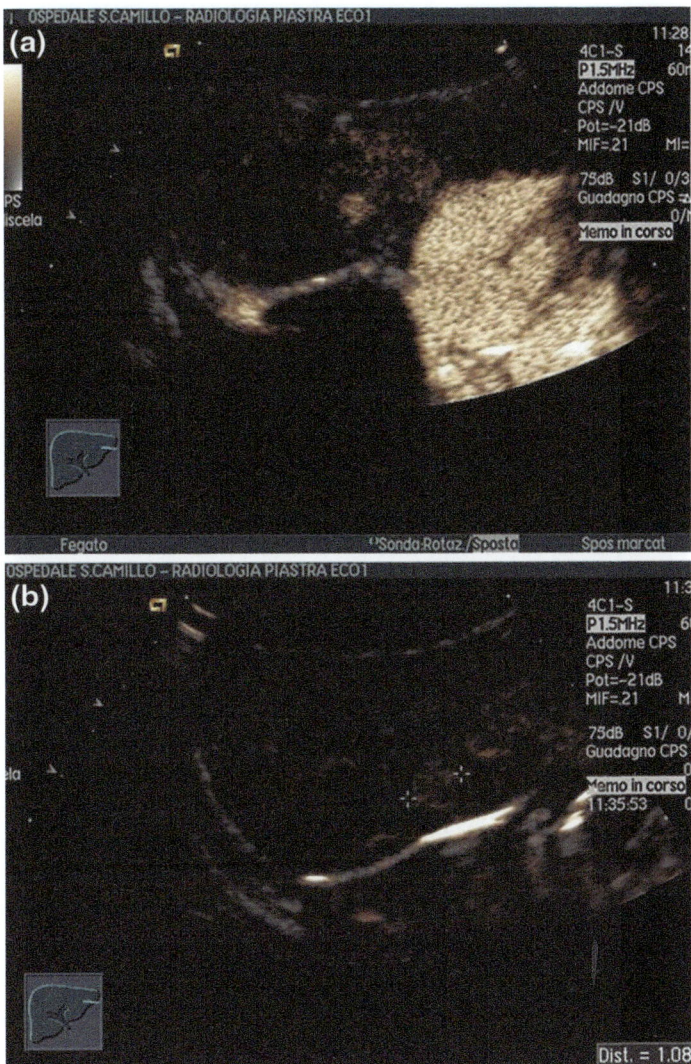

Fig. 4.9 **a–b** CEUS image of the findings identified in the baseline examination, which demonstrates a pattern typical of angiomas

In agreement with the parents and the pediatrician, we performed a contrast-enhanced ultrasound. The solid nodules showed early enhancement, which remained in the late-venous phase, showing the typical behavior of angiomas (Fig. 4.9a, b). Also, using ultrasound the nodules could be observed continuously for several minutes, unlike in the three individual steps involved with CT or MRI techniques. The subsequent standard ultrasound check-ups, completed after 3

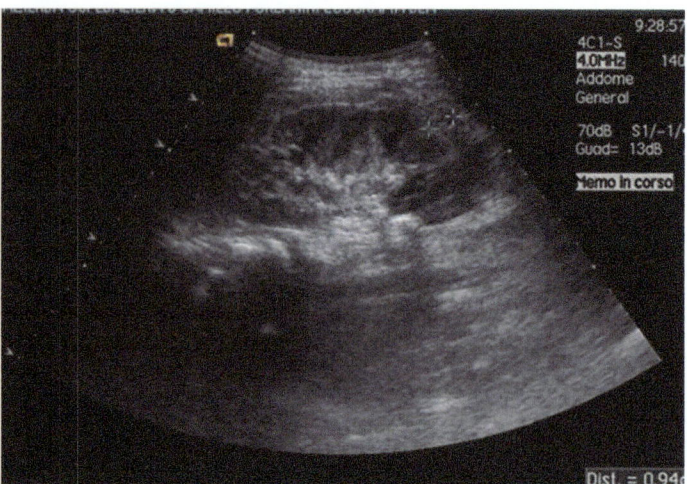

Fig. 4.10 Ultrasound baseline of a child with minor trauma but with hematuria: suspected lacerated-contusive lesion on the lower third of the right kidney

weeks, 2 months and 6 months, showed a gradual reduction of the angiomas, until they disappeared after a year and a half.

The second clinical case was a child with recent trauma and suspected hematoma in the baseline renal sonogram (Fig. 4.10). After contrast, the parenchymal laceration appeared with greater certainty, in the form of a clear nonvascularized space (Fig. 4.11), in both the venous and late phases.

In similar cases, contrast-enhanced examination has been very useful in reaching a diagnosis and avoiding more invasive tests for children.

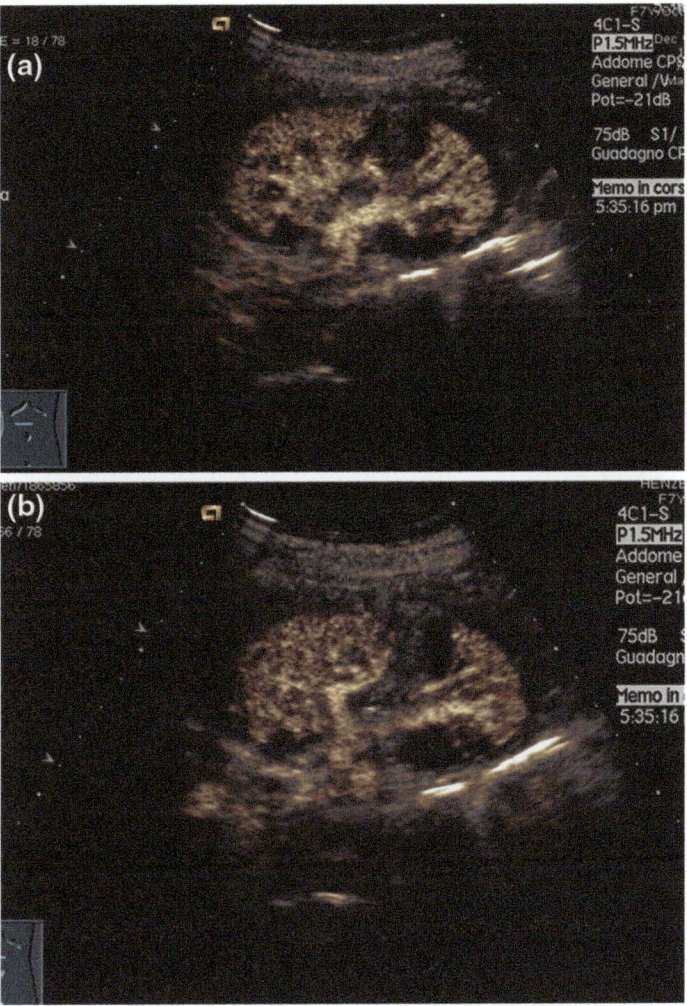

Fig. 4.11 a–b The CEUS clearly displays the presence of an avascular zone in a cortico medullary position, which points to an intraparenchymal contusion

References

1. Berrocal T, Gayá F, Arjonilla A, Lonergan GJ (2001) Vesicoureteral reflux: diagnosis and grading with echo-enhanced cystosonography versus voiding cystourethrography. Radiology 221:359–365
2. Claudon M, Cosgrove D, Albrecht T et al (2008) Guidelines and good clinical practice recommendations for contrast-enhanced ultrasound (CEUS), update 2008. Ultraschall Med 29:28–44

3. Darge K (2008) Voiding urosonography with ultrasound contrast agents for the diagnosis of vesicoureteric reflux in children. Pediatr Radiol 38(1):40–53
4. Darge K (2010) Voiding urosonography with US contrast agent for the diagnosis of vesicoureteric reflux in children: an update. Pediatr Radiol 40(6):956–962
5. Esposito F, Di Serafino M, Mercogliano F et al (2012) Ultrasound contrast media in paediatric patients: is it an off-label use? Regulatory requirements and radiologist's liability. Radiol Med 117:148–159
6. Faizah M, Kanaheswari Y, Thambidorai C, Zulfiqar M (2011) Echocontrast cystosonography versus micturating cystourethrography in the detection of vesicoureteric reflux. Biomed Imaging Interv J 7:e7
7. McCarville MB (2008) New frontiers in pediatric oncologic imaging. Cancer Imaging 8(1):87–92. Published online 25 March 2008. doi: 10.1102/1470-7330.2008.0012 PMCID: PMC2324372 9
8. Miele V, Buffa V, Stasolla A et al (2004) Contrast enhanced ultrasound with second generation contrast agent in traumatic liver lesions. Radiol Med 108:82–91
9. Otukesh H, Hoseini R, Behzadi AH et al (2011) Accuracy of cystosonography in the diagnosis of vesicourethral reflux in children. J Kidney Dis Transpl 22:488–491
10. Piscaglia F, Nolsøe C, Dietrich CF et al (2012) The EFSUMB guidelines and recommendations on the clinical practice of contrast enhanced ultrasound (CEUS): update 2011 on non-hepatic applications. Ultraschall Med 33:33–59
11. Riccabona M, Avni FE, Blickman JG et al (2008) Imaging recommendations in paediatric uroradiology: minutes of the ESPR workgroup session on urinary tract infection, fetal hydronephrosis, urinary tract ultrasonography and voiding cystourethrography, Barcelona, Spain, June 2007. Pediatr Radiol 38(2):138–145
12. Valentino M, Serra C, Pavlica P et al (2008) Blunt abdominal trauma: diagnostic performance of contrast enhanced US in children—initial experience. Radiology 246:903–909

Conclusions

5

The use of CEUS is to be considered, in such applications as the evaluation of ischemic and traumatic lesions and the characterization of cystic lesions, as a level II exam even with the currently most-commonly used imaging techniques, such as CT and MRI; and according to some authors, CEUS presents an even higher diagnostic accuracy.

Conversely, for the characterization of solid renal lesions and the detection of urothelial lesions, especially those of the upper urinary tract, it seems advisable to use further evaluation; in the first case, active semiquantitative software acts to evaluate the time/intensity curves; while, in the second case, uroCT scan is clearly favored. Bladder lesions may, according to some authors, benefit from the use of contrast ultrasound, especially when integrated with the baseline examination; but MRI using diffusion sequences currently appear to be superior in detection and in the evaluation of the T parameter.

It appears to be, based on our experience, an application that should be made mainstream and accepted as a first testing methodology in the evaluation of reflux in children; going beyond the current off-label use in this field and raising the awareness of governing bodies at both the hospital administrative and the ministerial level; the latter in order to fill a legislative gap that can no longer be tolerated and that continues to leave the diagnostician in a position of great difficulty from an procedural, but also moral standpoint.

G. Regine et al., *Contrast-Enhanced Ultrasound of the Urinary Tract*,
DOI: 10.1007/978-88-470-5432-5_5, © Springer-Verlag Italia 2013